ALLERGIES AND INFECTIOUS DISEASES

MEDIASTINAL INFECTIONS

CLINICAL DIAGNOSIS, SURGICAL AND ALTERNATIVE TREATMENTS

ALLERGIES AND INFECTIOUS DISEASES

Additional books in this series can be found on Nova's website under the Series tab.

Additional e-books in this series can be found on Nova's website under the e-book tab.

ALLERGIES AND INFECTIOUS DISEASES

MEDIASTINAL INFECTIONS

CLINICAL DIAGNOSIS, SURGICAL AND ALTERNATIVE TREATMENTS

WALID LEONARDO DAJER-FADEL
EDITOR

New York

Library of Congress Cataloging-in-Publication Data

ISBN: 978-1-63463-369-7

Library of Congress Control Number: 2014954112

Published by Nova Science Publishers, Inc. † New York

to my parents Leonardo and Daad for their never-ending support, and to my mentors Carlos Ibarra-Pérez, Rubén Argüero-Sánchez and Luis M. Argote-Greene who have served me as an example in my search for continued personal and professional improvement

Contents

Preface

In this book of *Mediastinal infections*, an amalgam of the most challenging clinical scenarios in infectious processes originated from the cervical, sternal or sub-diaphragmatic regions are analyzed in the field of thoracic and cardiac surgery. Since the discovery of drainage and lavage of infected spaces, a true battle against microorganisms has developed, the principles have not changed much over the years, however thanks to new technological advances, physicians have been gaining terrain when treating these patients. In the first chapter a thorough review of the key anatomical aspects that promote mediastinal infections is done, for many surgeons this is an intricate group of fascia and spaces that communicate the cervical with mediastinal regions, for that reason the authors did had a challenging task trying to simplify in a way easy to understand for the reader through diagrams and tomographic images. Since sepsis is the culprit of most demises, it was necessary to explore the ins and outs that produce and perpetuate the infectious process that overwhelms the body in a situation such as this, helping understand treatment protocols described in further chapters. By far, deep neck infections are to take the blame when an acute descending necrotizing mediastinitis (DNM) takes place, in this chapter a more specific view of the cervical anatomy is done before understanding the mechanisms and etiologies that produce this dreadful disease, pointing out the best evidence available for medical and surgical treatments offered in these cases. Immediately after, four chapters take the reader through an overview of DNM, the correlation between radiologic studies to diagnose and follow up on these patients, also a description of all the techniques done in the past for such an infection, to conclude with the medical treatment's perspective on the matter, approaching this illness from every possible angle often necessary to really understand what is happening from the structural, microbiological and metabolically point of view to adequately treat this pathology.

Ascending necrotizing mediastinitis, although rare, is included in this book since it also comprises a source of mediastinal infection, embryological facts are pointed out, as well as a recompilation of the scarce reports available in the literature, so management of these patients could be better understood.

Post-operative mediastinitis is discussed in the following four chapters, offering an overview of the disease, followed by a well explained analysis on correlative radiological anatomy for the diagnosis, because in these cases, this is the hardest aspect when trying to decide whether to operate or treat conservatively; it is followed by an excellent illustrated description of the surgical techniques and their indications, to finally conclude with a chapter on medical management, which is usually done at the cardiac Intensive Care Unit.

The last chapter centers its attention on the chronic causes of mediastinitis, where pathophysiology is explained, as well as the accurate diagnostic tools to perform an appropriate treatment plan.

We would like to acknowledge Heidy Higuera Hernández for the excellent illustrations throughout the book. We truly hope you enjoy reading this work.

In: Mediastinal Infections
Editor: Walid Leonardo Dajer-Fadel
ISBN: 978-1-63463-369-7

Chapter 1

Anatomy of the Neck and Mediastinum, the Principles of Infection

W. L. Dajer-Fadel[1,*] ***and C. Ibarra-Pérez***[2]
[1]Cardiothoracic Surgery Department,
General Hospital of Mexico "Dr. Eduardo Liceaga",
Mexico City, Mexico
[2]National Academy of Medicine, Mexico City,
Mexico

Abstract

The mediastinum harvests some of the most vital organs, therefore when fighting against infectious processes, knowledge of their relations with fascia and spaces of the neck, infra-abdominal viscera and superficial thoracic planes are of the outmost importance for the thoracic surgeon, clinician and radiologist; this has been a difficult subject to explain throughout the years since education about it has always been done in a superficial way during medical school and residency, the goal of this chapter is to present it in an easy to understand format, in a way that makes sense for the reader. A review of the anatomical configuration of the neck, mediastinum and the relation between them, clarifying the pathways from which infections can extend from above, below and

* Correspondence to: drdajer@gmail.com.

superficially. Also, the anatomical landmarks that the surgeon needs to know in order to adequately locate the site of incision when an infection ensues. Finally it will analyze the theories on how microorganisms have the advantage when spreading from a site outside of the thoracic cavity, into it. A flow diagram is offered to explain all the points discussed in the chapter, from the sites of origin up until reaching the mediastinal spaces, correlating it with the pathways of spread for disease.

Introduction

It is essential to understand the anatomical aspects of these infectious processes; the mediastinum is the final stop for many sites of origin, such as: the cervical region and its corresponding spaces and fascia, the upper thoracic skin, the sternum and the infra-diaphragmatic regions. Each type of infection carries a particular pathophysiology and it is of the outmost importance to have it clear in the physician's mind at the time of diagnostic workup. When infections propagate, an interesting correlation exists between the sites of origin and the final destination, understanding this is the first step in a tortuous pathway towards success in the management of patients that arrive to the ER or that are being treated at any ICU. For the unexperienced eye, it's just the tip of the iceberg and carries a great burden to the thoracic surgeon when fighting against the most feared result, a mediastinal infection followed by death. In this chapter we are going to review and discuss the anatomical principles from an apparently mild infection until it reaches a full blown mediastinitis.

Cervical Anatomy, Fascia and Spaces

The anatomical principles of the neck´s base and thoracic inlet that are usually thought, are originally taken from standard textbooks, this may not be the ideal scenario to one´s knowledge on the subject, since specialists need to have another perspective on the matter, because of the complex structural arrangement of arteries, veins, muscles and most importantly, spaces and fascia. [1]

The identifiable skin landmarks of the neck are noted by the laryngeal prominence (Adam´s apple) formed by the apex of the "V" shape formed by the two laminae of the thyroid cartilage at the level of C_4-C_5. The cricoid cartilage (at the level of C_6) lies inferior to the prominence, followed caudally by the 18-22 "C" shaped cartilages that form the trachea; the thyroid gland lies at the level of the 2nd and 3rd cartilaginous rings in front and laterally of the proximal trachea, which is crossed in the midline by its isthmus. Attached to this airway, on the external surface, lies the pre-tracheal fascia, identified when performing a tracheotomy. [1]

Important muscles in this area are the prevertebral, scalene, sternocleidomastoid, platysma and the trapezius muscles which give strength to the neck and surrounding structures, in many instances they play a role in incision decisions regarding neck and mediastinal drainage for the treatment of mediastinitis, mostly the descending necrotizing type. [1]

The fascial planes and spaces are considered the culprit when analyzing the ways infectious processes spread to the mediastinum; the following are the most important structures that favor microbial advancement:

Submandibular space: Located between the submandibular and submentonian triangles, between the mucosa of the oral cavity´s floor and superficial layer of the deep cervical fascia; it is divided by the mylohyoid muscle, in a *sublingual space,* which contains the sublingual gland, hypoglosal nerve, part of the submandibular gland, and loose connective tissue; and the *submylohyoid space,* which contains the submandibular salivary glands; both spaces are communicated posteriorly, around the mylohyoid muscle.

Parapharyngeal space: Also known as the lateral pharyngeal space, located in the lateral aspect of the neck in the shape of an inverted cone, with the skull as the base and apex as the hyoid bone, it is immersed in the pharyngeal constrictor muscle, medially contiguous to the pre-tracheal fascia of the visceral zone, laterally with the superficial fascia (which surrounds the parotid gland), pterygoid muscle and mandible. It is subdivided in anterior and posterior compartments, the first only contains lymph nodes, muscle, adipose and connective tissue, which are in direct relation to the tonsillar fossa and the internal pterygoid muscle. The posterior compartment contains cranial nerves IX and XII, carotid sheath with its contents, and the cervical sympathetic trunk; the carotid sheath, found in the posterior section of the para-pharyngeal space, perforates the connus in its apex to enter the mediastinum. Infections of the parapharyngeal space could be due to tonsillitis, pharyngitis, mumps, otitis or mastoiditis and finally, infections of odontogenic origin (Ludwig´s angina).

Retropharyngeal and *prevertebral (between the prevertebral fascia and the vertebral bodies) spaces:* Lined anteriorly by the constrictor muscles of the neck and posteriorly by the superficial layer of the deep cervical fascia. Located behind the hypopharynx and esophagus, communicating with the parapharyngeal space laterally where the carotid sheath is found; this space includes the "dangerous space" (between the alar and prevertebral fascia) which is located posterior to the retropharyngeal space, it extends from the base of the skull and freely descends throughout the mediastinum behind the diaphragm (T1 – T2) where both fascia meet providing the most important route for dissemination of a mediastinal infection. It also includes the prevertebral space that is surrounded by the prevertebral fascia, it extends from the base of the skull until it reaches the coccyx, allowing microorganisms to propagate as low as the psoas´ aponeurosis (Figure 1).

Superficial (investing) fascia: It encircles the neck in its totality, attached superiorly to the superior nuchal line and spinous processes of C_1-C_7 and inferiorly to the manubrium, clavicle and scapula, in its superior portion this fascia splits into two layers which attach to the anterior and posterior manubrium harvesting the suprasternal space (or space of Burns) containing the sternal heads of the sternocleidomastoid muscles and the arch of the internal jugular vein.

Middle (pretracheal) fascia: Extends from the thyroid and cricoid cartilages down into the thorax which splits to surround the thyroid gland, trachea and esophagus in a complete pattern. This fascia includes the strap muscles which eventually fuse with the superficial fascia opposite to the carotid sheath, in cases of spontaneous pneumomediastinum, air reaches the neck dissecting along these planes in 14.5% of the cases.

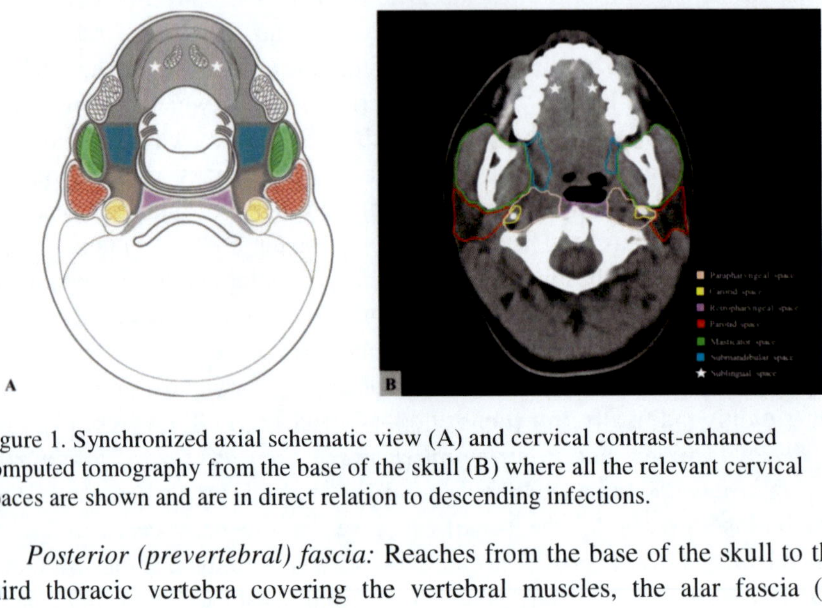

Figure 1. Synchronized axial schematic view (A) and cervical contrast-enhanced computed tomography from the base of the skull (B) where all the relevant cervical spaces are shown and are in direct relation to descending infections.

Posterior (prevertebral) fascia: Reaches from the base of the skull to the third thoracic vertebra covering the vertebral muscles, the alar fascia (or prevertebral fascia) lies posterior to the visceral compartment of the neck continuing to form the carotid sheath which could also be a way for descending infections. [2, 3] The pretracheal space, located behind the strap muscles is seen during a mediastinoscopy, thyroid surgery or surgery of the cervical tracheal; also serves as the site for drainage during the cervical phase of descending necrotizing mediastinitis, extending from the thyroid cartilage to the upper part of the aortic arch where the pericardium attaches superiorly to this artery, limiting infectious spread downwards.

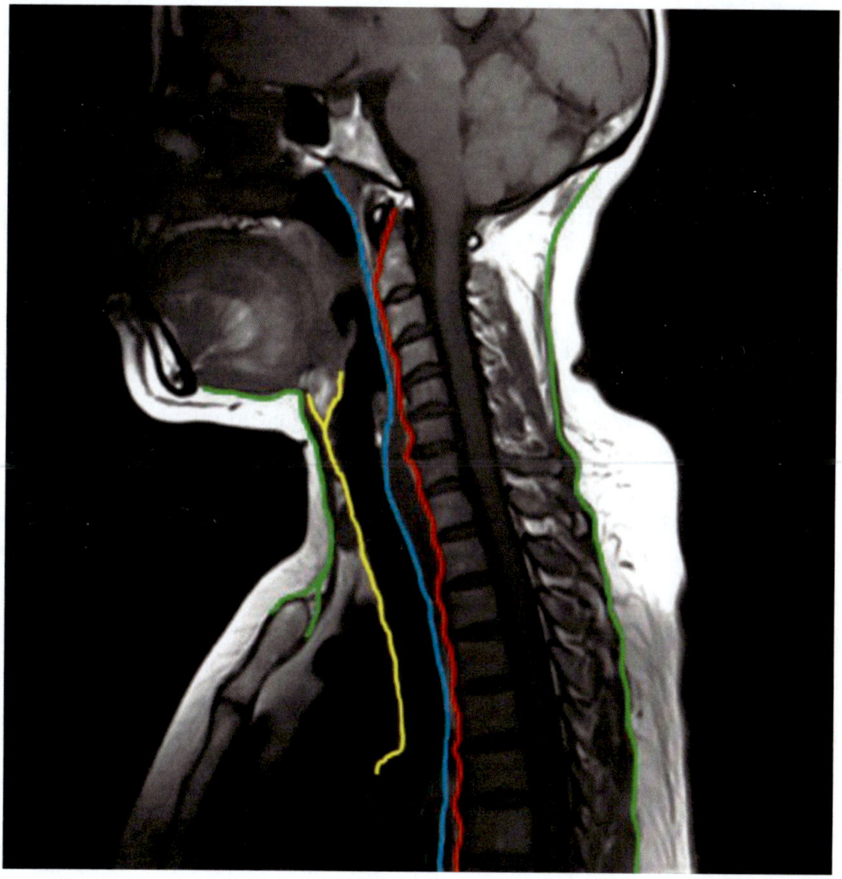

Figure 2. Sagittal T1-weighted magnetic resonance image explaining the relation between the fascia of the neck and mediastinum through the pretracheal (*yellow*), buccopharyngeal (*blue*), prevertebral (*red*) and the investing (*green*) fascia.

The retrovisceral or retropharyngeal space is formed by loose connective tissue that lies in front of the prevertebral fascia reaching the diaphragm (Figure 2). [1]

Mediastinal Anatomy

The mediastinum is an area limited in the superior region by the thoracic inlet, inferiorly by the diaphragm, anteriorly by the internal surface of the sternum, posteriorly by the longitudinal spinal ligament and vertebral spine, finally in its lateral aspects, by the mediastinal pleura of both sides; strictly speaking the costovertebral sulci are not included, however, many times they are considered when tumors originate from these spaces. The mediastinum contains vital structures that cannot be overlooked by the thoracic surgeons when treating patients with infections in these regions, among these, are the heart, great arteries and veins, trachea, esophagus and others, such as the thoracic duct and nerves.

Historically, the anatomical boundaries of its spaces have been a subject of debate to understand, classify and plan surgical interventions for infected patients, to unify and reach universal criteria; unfortunately, a consensus has not been reached so we will discuss the most relevant propositions and finally suggest our most comprehensive view for the surgeon regarding mediastinal infections.

Gray [4] in his original anatomy text, first described the compartments as superior, anterior, middle and posterior. The superior is located above an imaginary line traced from Louis´ angle to C_4, anteriorly in front of the pericardium, middle contained by the pericardium and posterior everything that lies behind the pericardium, although easy to understand we believe it to be inaccurate from a surgeon´s perspective when treating mediastinal infections. Years after, other classifications emerged with a tricompartamental model suggesting an anterior (antero-superior), middle and posterior compartments. [5-6] Other proposals exist subdividing the mediastinum in six compartments which result complex and useless for the clinicians and surgeons alike. [7]

Our consensus supports Shields´ [8] proposal which is conceptually, anatomically and surgically sound, modifying the location of the three compartments in zones as *prevascular* (anterior), *visceral* (middle) and *retrovisceral* (which contains the costovertebral sulci) that are clearly visible in radiographic studies (Figure 3).

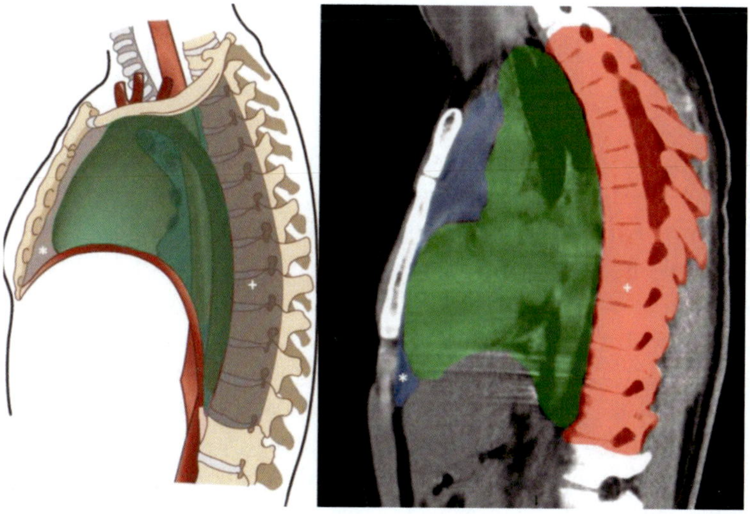

Figure 3. Synchronized schematic left lateral (A) and (B) sagittal simple tomographic views of the chest showing the prevascular (*asteriks*), visceral (*green*) and retrovisceral (*plus signs*) zones of Shields.

This model is also used for mediastinal tumors to identify the origin of the mass which is defined by the majority of its occupying area and not the site where it grew from.

The *prevascular zone* extends anteriorly from the internal surface of the sternum, superiorly by the innominate artery and veins, posteriorly by an imaginary line formed by the anterior surface of the pericardium and great arteries and veins, and inferiorly delimitated by the diaphragm; it contains lymphatic nodes from the sternal groups, anterior mediastinum, and connective and adipose tissues; it is also possible to find ectopic parathyroid glands and thyroid tissue where the most common anterior mediastinal masses, such as neoplasms of the thymus, germ cell tumors, retrosternal thyroid, lymphomas and bronchogenic cysts are found; it also presents as a reservoir for purulent exudates and anterior mediastinal infections, mostly seen in post-operative and some descending necrotizing mediastinitis.

The *visceral zone* occupies all the structures of the thoracic inlet; superiorly limited by the innominate artery and veins behind the sternum, extending underneath these structures, posterior to the *prevascular zone* in the anterior surface of the pericardium, its posterior boundary is limited by the longitudinal spinal ligament, ventral to the spinal column; within this space lies the pericardium, heart, great arteries and veins, trachea, proximal portion of right and left bronchii, supra-aortic arteries, para-aortic surface, esophagus, lymphatic nodes, vagus nerve, different plexus and nerve fibers, thoracic duct, proximal azygos vein, and connective and adipose tissue. The most common masses found in this zone are lymphomas, bronchogenic, esophageal, neuroenteric and pericardial cysts, also lung neoplasms that invade the mediastinum; paradoxically being the most ample compartment of the mediastinum, mediastinal infections are rarely found in this space, when this occurs, its mostly related to infections extending from the carotid sheath.

In regards to the *retrovisceral zone*, which contains the costovertebral sulci and its direct relation to the prevertebral fascia and retroesophageal space, serves as the origin for masses that grow and protrude from this region; also allowing superior infections to reach the mediastinum and provoke a full blown septic state. It contains proximal portions of intercostal arteries and veins, the proximal segment of the anterior and communicating ramus of intercostal nerves, thoracic spinal ganglia, sympathetic trunk and its branches, connective and lymphatic tissue, and the distal azygos vein. This zone´s tumors are characterized according to the structure that originated them, such is the case of the intercostal nerve, producing neurofibromas, neurilemmomas (Schwannomas), neurofibrosarcoma and neurosarcoma, the ones originated from sympathetic ganglia such as ganglioneuroma, ganglioneuroblastoma and neuroblastoma; the ones originated from paraganglionar cells such as paraganglioma (pheochromocytomas); and rarely, lymphomas are seen in this zone. In the pediatric population neurogenic tumors are the most frequent, in approximately half of this population. As said before, this is the most common landing zone for mediastinal infections of the descending type, in most situations these propagate from the retro-pharyngeal into the retro-esophageal space dissecting and containing large volumes of purulent exudate, this is the most important space that needs to be drained during surgical treatment for these infections. [9-11]

Anatomical Landmarks of Importance for Neck and Mediastinal Infections

Topographical landmarks are often a neglected part of teaching in surgical practice, maybe because more often than not, it is inferred that the trainee dominates this knowledge, however it is often evidenced in daily practice that this is far from true. For this reason the authors believe this must be included in the chapter, to better understand the relationship of surface features to deeper structures as an invaluable tool in the clinical assessment of a patient and for the interpretation of radiologic imaging. With this in mind, familiarity with these thoracic landmarks will serve as a prerequisite for understanding and applying adequate placement of thoracic and neck incisions for the treatment of mediastinal infectious processes.

To start off, the muscular landmarks are as follow, the sternocleidomastoid originated by two heads from the manubrium and the medial head of the clavicle extend diagonally upwards onto the mastoid process at the base of the skull. The medial border, easily seen when the patient´s head faces laterally, serves as a landmark for cervical incisions, used to approach the esophagus and the spaces of the vicinity, and the jugular vein. The pectoralis major muscle extends from the second to sixth costal cartilages and ribs, sternum and medial half of the clavicle passing as a fan-shaped muscle to insert into the intertubercular groove of the humerus, the lateral border corresponds to the anterior fold of the axilla, in men the lower border translates to the fifth rib. Below this muscle, lies the serratus anterior muscle on the antero-lateral aspect of the chest wall, which rises from the muscular slips of the first eight ribs reaching the vertebral border of the scapula, its highest visible digitation on thin patients is associated to the sixth rib (Figure 4). In the posterior aspect of the thorax, lies the latissimus dorsi, the most important reference muscle for the thoracic surgeon, originated from a broad aponeurosis of the lower six thoracic vertebra, the lumbodorsal fascia, and the iliac crest to finally extend in to the intertubercular groove, in its lateral side, forms the posterior fold of the axilla. Once this is understood, it is easy to identify the axillary lines, since the anterior line is recognized by its anterior fold, the posterior line is originated from the posterior fold and finally the mid-axillary line is placed between these two. The fourth intercostal space is easily identified in men by the nipple in the mid-clavicular line (Figure 5). [12]

The bones are also of great importance to identify internal structures, the manubrium defines the suprasternal notch in its upper border, used to perform a mediastinoscopy, tracheotomy or collar incisions, also corresponds to the first thoracic spinous process or second thoracic vertebra, it also overlies the aortic arch; in its inferior border when articulating with the sternal body forming Louis´ angle, palpable in most patients where the second rib invariably articulates, it also corresponds to the fourth thoracic vertebra and the tracheal carina, also parallel to the right of this structure lies the azygos vein reaching the superior vena cava, finally, this is the site where the thoracic duct crosses from right to left in front of the vertebral column. The sternal body, corresponds to $T_5 - T_9$ vertebral bodies (Figure 4).

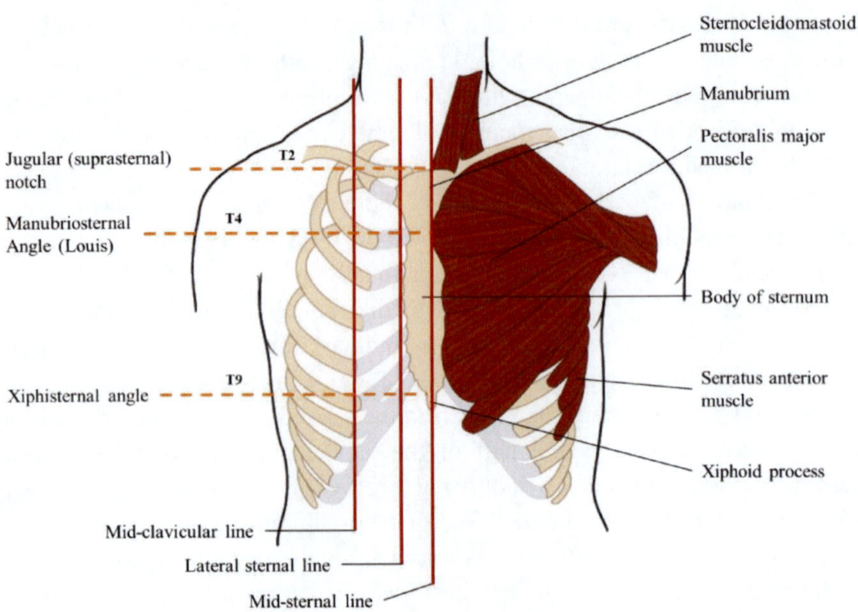

Figure 4. Anterior view demonstrating the topographical lines for reference to internal viscera.

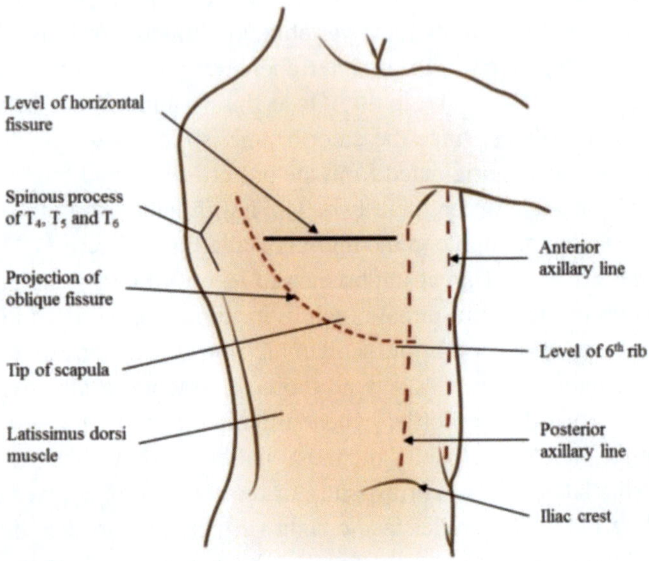

Figure 5. Lateral view demonstrating the topographical lines for reference to internal viscera.

Anatomical and Physiological Principles for the Origin of Mediastinal Infections

In figure 6, the main pathways of infection are depicted, it is hypothesized that propagation of infectious processes in descending necrotizing mediastinitis are favored by several factors: a) negative pressure from the thoracic cavity (which usually oscillates between -5 and -10 cmH_2O), b) gravity and c) gas producing microorganisms that dissect through the fascial planes and spaces allowing them to advance towards the mediastinal compartments.

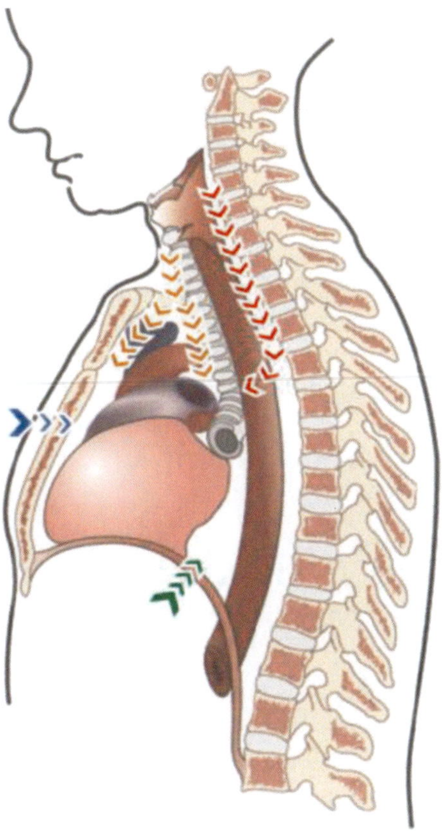

Figure 6. Schematic representation infectious spread in acute mediastinal infections demonstrating the descending (*orange and red arrows*), post-operative (*blue arrows*) and ascending (*green arrows*) types.

However, no scientific work is available proving these points; it makes sense after observing the way this disease develops in the descending type. In some cases the infection spreads from the skin or bony structures as reported in the past. When this happens, invasion occurs in such an overwhelming fashion and velocity that medical treatment is not effective, allowing the disease to spread to deep fascia, advancing by contiguity until reaching the mediastinum. [13-16] For the post-operative type, the explanation is straight forward, direct invasion generally occurs from the surgical wound that gets out of medical control, advances to Camper´s fascia which is in direct contact with the sternum, when this bone is affected, osteomyelitis ensues, once this point is reached it becomes harder to treat as it will be discussed in future chapters; at this point, if medical treatment has not been successful or the disease not identified, it will continue inward provoking mediastinal invasion. Other anatomical factors influence this reduced protection against infection i.e., harvesting the internal thoracic arteries originated from the subclavian arteries running 1.5 – 2.5 cm parallel from each sternal border, used for coronary artery bypass surgery, reducing vascular flow, therefore oxygenation and white blood cell availability of the infected area.

For the ascending type, although very rare, it is believed that tracking or invasion through the esophageal and aortic hiatuses are one of the main pathways of infection, summoned to the intra-thoracic negative pressure and in some instances direct structural relation of intra-abdominal structures to the diaphragm, allowing upward flow of microorganisms to the mediastinum. Also as mentioned before, the prevertebral fascia which extends until it reaches the coccyx could play a role in this type. [17, 18]

Vascular Considerations of the Mediastinum

The thoracic cavity is one of the most susceptible regions of the body, prone to devastating septic processes when it comes to infections, in great measure, it is believed to be due to the a large vascular and lymphatic network that play a role in the overwhelming inflammatory response that takes place during mediastinitis. Just as a reminder, thoracic wall supply is done by the intercostal arteries which are formed by an anastomosis of their posterior and anterior counterparts. The posterior intercostal arteries have their origin in all (except the first two) spaces from the posterior aortic wall; the first two originate from the superior intercostal artery, a branch of the costo-cervical trunk. These arteries give off collateral branches supplying the posterior and lateral portions of their corresponding spaces. The upper 6 anterior intercostal arteries are originated from the internal thoracic artery and the remaining four spaces receive arteries from the musculophrenic artery (a branch of the mammary arteries). Also, the upper two intercostal spaces are supplied by the supreme thoracic artery (branch of the axillary artery), these travel above and beyond each rib anteriorly. Veins have a similar pattern of distribution draining to the azygos system and brachiocephalic veins.

Bronchial arteries originate from the antero-lateral parts of the descending aorta between the level of T_5 and T_6 vertebra, it is important that the surgeon is aware that this anatomy is very variable. In the majority of cases, a right bronchial artery (RBA) originates from the first ipsilateral intercostal artery, called "intercosto-bronchial artery"; the RBA has a length of 5 -8 cm giving branches to the esophagus in its mid-portion, the trachea, the pericardium, left atrium, mediastinal lymph nodes, vessels and nerves (specially the vagus); at the level of the main bronchus, it divides in its carinal portion, the upper lobe, the intermediary bronchus and lower lobe. The left is usually irrigated by two arteries, their length varies from 2 to 4.5 cm, almost always originating from the anterior aortic wall directed towards the upper and lower lobes. [19-22]

It is important to note that this anatomy varies all the time, however, the importance of chest wall and mediastinal irrigation make this a sensible subject when analyzing mediastinal infections.

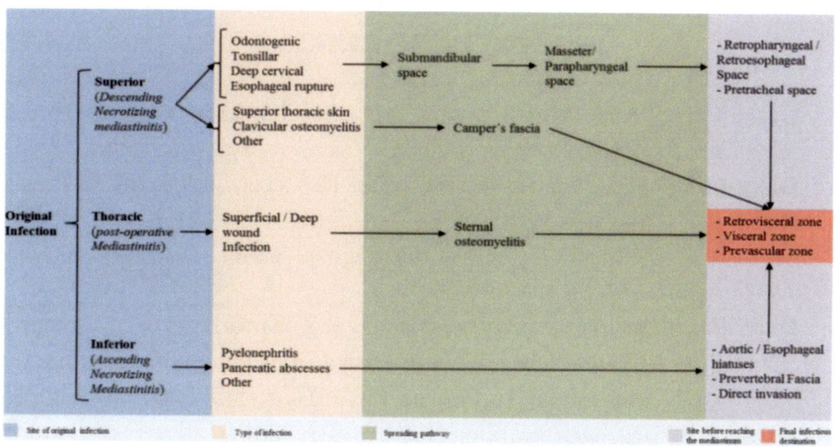

Figure 7. Flow diaphragm showing how and through which pathways mediastinal infections develop as time lapses without successful medical treatment.

Cardiopulmonary circulation is of little importance when considering mediastinitis. Lymphatic circulation within the mediastinum is worth mentioning when considering a septic process of this area, it is usually divided in collectors of the lower and upper mediastinum; in general the lymph node chains drain from both lungs and mediastinal viscera, it is an intricate system where also nodes from the pericardium and anterior mediastinum are involved. It is common to find enlarged nodes in CT scans of patients with mediastinitis; also, infection has been reported after punctured necrotic nodes by transesophageal endoscopic ultrasound with fine-needle aspiration. [22, 23]

Conclusion

As explained throughout the chapter, having a clear understanding of the thoracic anatomy is primordial for planning any surgical approach for the treatment of mediastinitis, various factors play a role in the propagation of this disease from an anatomical and physiological point of view, for ease of understanding an algorithm (Figure 7) is presented signaling all the important anatomical features derived from different points of origin as they evolve to a mediastinal infection. In future chapters knowledge of the normal anatomy is essential to understand the surgical procedures explained throughout the book for the treatment of the three kinds of acute mediastinal infections.

References

[1] Deslauriers J. Anatomy of the neck and cervicothoracic junction. *Thorac Surg Clin* 2007;17:529-547.

[2] Dajer-Fadel W. L., Ibarra-Pérez C., Sánchez-Velázquez L. D., Borrego-Borrego R., Navarro-Reynoso F. P., Argüero-Sánchez R. Descending necrotizing mediastinitis below the tracheal carina. *Asian Cardiovasc Thorac Ann* 2014;22(2):176-182.

[3] Dajer-Fadel W. L., Argüero-Sánchez R., Ibarra-Pérez C., Navarro-Reynoso F. P. Systematic review of spontaneous pneumomediastinum: a survey of 22 years' data. *Asian Cardiovasc Thorac Ann* 2014;22(8): 997-1002.

[4] Gray H. Gray´s Anatomy: The anatomical basis of medicine and surgery. Ed. 38. New York: Churchill Livingstone; 1995.

[5] Whitten C. R., Khan S., Munneke G. J., et al. A diagnostic approach to mediastinal abnormalities. *Radiographics* 2007;27:657-671.

[6] Zylak C. J., Paillic W., Jackson R. Correlative anatomy and computed tomography: a module on the mediastinum. *Radiographics* 1982;2:555-592.

[7] Heitzman E. R. The mediastinum: radiologic correlation with anatomy and pathology. Ed. 1. St. Louis (MO): Mosby; 1997. Pp. 216-234.

[8] Shields T. W. Primary tumors and cysts of the mediastinum. General Thoracic Surgery. Ed. 1. Philadelphia: Lea and Febiger; 1972. p. 908.

[9] Takeda S., Miyoshi S., Akashi A., et al. Clinical spectrum of primary mediastinal tumors: a comparison of adult and pediatric populations at a single Japanese institution. *J Surg Oncol* 2003;83:24-30.

[10] Mullen B., Richardson J. D. Primary anterior mediastinal tumors in children and adults. *Ann Thorac Surg* 1986;42:338-345.

[11] Dajer-Fadel W. L., Ibarra-Pérez C., Argüero-Sánchez R. Mediastinal drainage in descending necrotizing mediastinitis. *Asian Cardiovasc Thorac Ann* 2013;21(4):493-495.

[12] Sayeed R. A., Darling G. E. Surface anatomy and Surface landmarks for thoracic surgery. *Thorac Surg Clin* 2007;17:449-461.

[13] Dajer-Fadel W. L., Ibarra-Pérez C., Borrego-Borrego R., Flores-Calderón O. Thoracic necrotizing fasciitis due to snake ointment that progressed to a mediastinitis. *Interact Cardiovasc Thorac Surg* 2012;14(1):94–95.

[14] Dajer-Fadel W. L., Ibarra-Pérez C., Borrego-Borrego R., Navarro-Reynoso F. P., Argüero-Sánchez R. Descending necrotizing mediastinitis and sternoclavicular joint osteomyelitis. *Asian Cardiovasc Thorac Ann* 2013;21(5):618-620.

[15] Dajer-Fadel W. L., Borrego-Borrego R., Flores-Calderon O., Ibarra-Perez C. Descending necrotizing mediastinitis and thoracic cellulitis due to varicella. *Asian Cardiovasc Thorac Ann* 2012;20(1):83-85.

[16] Cirino L. M., Elias F. M., Almeida J. L. Descending mediastinitis: a review. *Sao Paulo Med J* 2006;124:285-290.

[17] Chang Y. C., Chen C. W. Thoracoscopic drainage of ascending mediastinitis arising from pancreatic pseudocyst. *Interact Cardiovasc Thorac Surg* 2009;9(1):144-145.

[18] Dajer-Fadel W. L., Pichardo-González M., Estrada-Ramos S., Palafóx D., Navarro-Reynoso F. P., Argüero-Sánchez R. Ascending necrotizing mediastinitis secondary to emphysematous pyelonephritis. *Asian Cardiovasc Thorac Ann* 2014;22(7):869-871.

[19] Remy-Jardin M., Bouaziz N., Dumont P., Brillet P. Y., Bruzzi J., Remy J. Bronchial and non bronchial systemic arteries at multidetector row CT angiography: comparison with conventional angiography. *Radiology* 2004;233:741–749.

[20] Carles J., Clerc F., Dubrez J., Couraud L., Drouillard J., Videau J. The bronchial arteries: anatomic study and application to lung transplantation. *Surg Radiol Anat* 1995;17:293–299.

[21] Schreinemakers H. H., Weder W., Miyoshi S., Harper B. D., Shimokawa S., Egan T. M., McKnight R., Cooper J. D. Direct revascularization of bronchial arteries for lung transplantation: an anatomical study. *Ann Thorac Surg* 1990;49:44–45.

[22] Riquet M. Bronchial arteries and lymphatics of the lung. *Thorac Surg Clin* 2007;17:619-638.

[23] Aerts J. G., Kloover J., Los J., van der Heijden O., Janssens A., Tournoy K. G. EUS-FNA of enlarged necrotic lymph nodes may cause infectious mediastinitis. *J Thorac Oncol* 2008;3(10):1191-1193.

In: Mediastinal Infections
Editor: Walid Leonardo Dajer-Fadel
ISBN: 978-1-63463-369-7

Chapter 2

Deep Neck Infections

***J. A. Solis-Suarez*[1,*] *and A. Carillo-Muñoz*[1]**
[1]Ear, Nose and Throat Department,
General Hospital of Mexico "Dr. Eduardo Liceaga",
Mexico City, Mexico

Abstract

Deep Neck Infections (DNI) are caused by bacteria that result in abscess or cellulitis in potential neck spaces, they can originate from several sources; the main ones are: odontogenic, followed by upper respiratory tract infections, intravenous drug abuse, sialoadenitis, sialolithiasis, paranasal sinuses, brachial sinuses and malignancies. Associated comorbidities such as diabetes mellitus and cardiovascular diseases play a very important role in disease progression, also are the growing number of patients with immune dysfunctions, which play an important role in morbidity and mortality. Knowledge of the anatomy is very important for diagnosis, management and treatment of complications. DNI appear as polymicrobial infections with aerobic and anaerobic bacteria, making initial treatment with empiric antibiotics imperative, also choosing the right surgical treatment to avoid fatal complications.

* E-mail: jsolis.orl@gmail.com.

Introduction

DNI are common and occur as a consequence of bacterial infections from de upper aero-digestive tract, but they have other several etiologies. The result is either an abscess or cellulitis in the potential –superficial or deep- spaces of the neck. There is not much information regarding the true incidence of these infections. Treatment has been based mostly on surgical principles, airway management, and an understanding of the microbiological flora. Today, neck infections are rarely life threatening when sound and timely management are applied. Nevertheless, mortality increases when some complications appear, such as descending mediastinitis, pericarditis, airway obstruction, pneumonia, pleural effusion, jugular vein thrombosis, septic shock and erosion of carotid artery. Infection with abscess or cellulitis typically spreads along fascial planes and potential spaces of the head and neck region; therefore, in order to treat them, there must be an extensive knowledge of the neck´s anatomy. It is of note that prevalence and complication incidence of DNI have diminished with improved diagnostic techniques, dental care and widespread availability of antimicrobial therapy.

Anatomy

All neck elements are included within the layers of cervical fascia, which compose the potential neck spaces; these are important factors to outline the spread of infection, so we must know the anatomy to do a correct diagnosis and treatment of DNI.

Cervical Fascial Planes

There are two main cervical fascia; the superficial cervical and the deep cervical, which is divided into three layers (superficial, middle, and deep) that envelop the contents of the head and neck forming the potential deep neck spaces. The superficial cervical fascia covers in its upper limit the adipose tissue, superficial blood vessels, lymph vessels, nerves and muscles of facial expression, as well as the platysma; its lower limit is marked by the shoulders.

The superficial layer of the deep cervical fascia has its upper limit at the zygomatic arches, its lower limit in the superior border of the sternum, the posterior insertions are the vertebral spinous processes and the anterior insertions are the hyoid and jaw bone. Within its contents are: the sternocleidomastoid, trapezius, masseter, anterior digastric muscles, and the parotid and submandibular salivary glands. Two virtual spaces are formed by the parotid and masticator spaces, contributing to the formation of the carotid space forming its lateral limit.

The middle layer of the deep cervical fascia has a subdivision, one covering muscular structures and the other, visceral structures, muscle division has its upper limit at the hyoid and lower limit in the clavicle and scapula, contains the sternothyroid, sternohyoid, and thyrohyoid muscles, the visceral subdivision has its upper boundary at the pharyngeal constrictor muscles and its lower limit at the mediastinal pre-vascular zone, overlying the fibrous pericardium and great vessels, covers the trachea, larynx, pharynx, esophagus, and thyroid gland. And it contributes to the formation of the antero-medial limit of the carotid space.

The deep cervical fascia´s layer contains the posterior structures of the neck, the anterior origin are the vertebral spinous processes and surrounds the posterior muscles of the neck and spine, it divides to form the alar fascia which forms the posterior wall of the retropharyngeal space and pre-vertebral fascia that's attached to the vertebral bodies forming the posterior wall of dangerous space, it covers the brachial plexus, phrenic nerves and vertebral blood vessels. It contributes to the creation of the carotid space lateral limit.

The carotid sheath receives contributions from all three layers of the deep cervical fascia, and still is a barrier against the spread of infection into the carotid space from the adjacent deep neck spaces.

Deep Neck Spaces

Deep neck spaces virtual are formed and delimited by the cervical fascia, there are potentially 11, that can be divided in 3 groups: suprahyoid, infrahyoid and total cervical.

Suprahyoid Spaces

Peritonsillar space: The peritonsillar space lies within the palatine tonsil, limited by the anterior and posterior tonsillar pillars, the upper limit is the pharyngeal constrictor muscle and contains areolar connective tissue.

Submandibular space: The submandibular space is limited superiorly by the floor of the mouth and the deep cervical´s superficial fascia, laterally by the mandibular body and inferiorly by the hyoid bone; the mylohyoid muscle divides the submaxilar and sublingual spaces, which communicate without any limitations.

It contains connective tissue, submandibular and sublingual glands, Wharton's duct, geniohyoid muscles, lingual and hypoglossal nerves, anterior belly of digastric muscles, and lymph nodes.

Parapharyngeal space: Located between the visceral division of the middle layer of deep cervical fascia medially and the superficial layer of deep cervical fascia, limited above by the base of the skull, inferiorly by the hyoid bone, medially by the pharyngeal constrictor muscle, laterally by the mandibular body and medial pterygoid muscles, posteriorly by the prevertebral fascia and anteriorly by the pterigomandibular raphe which is divided into two compartments by the styloid, stylohyoid, stylopharyngeus, and styloglossus muscles; the prestyloid compartment contains: the internal maxillary artery, maxillary nerve and adipose tissue; the poststyloid compartment contains: the carotid artery, internal jugular vein, cervical sympathetic chain, and cranial nerves IX, X, XI and XII.

Buccal space: Lies within the buccopharyngeal fascia; its medial limit is the buccinator muscle and its lateral one, the skin, limited inferiorly by the border of the mandible and posteriorly by the pterygomandibular raphe, it contains the buccal fat pad, Stenon`s Duct and the facial artery.

Parotid space: The capsule that forms the superficial layer of deep cervical fascia, which covers the parotid gland, forms the parotid space; the medial boundary is the parapharyngeal space, to which it can communicate directly.

It contains the parotid gland, facial nerve, external carotid artery, lymph nodes, and superficial auricular-temporal nerve.

Total Cervical Spaces

Retropharyngeal space: The retropharyngeal space, which is bounded anteriorly by the visceral fascia, found behind the pharynx and esophagus and posteriorly bound by the alar fascia, it extends from the base of the skull to the mediastinum at the level of the second thoracic vertebra, laterally is limited by the carotid sheaths, forming a central division that contains two lymph node chains.

Dangerous space: Limited anteriorly by the alar fascia and posteriorly by prevertebral fascia, extending from the skull´s base to the mediastinum at the level of the diaphragm.

Prevertebral space: The prevertebral space is limited anteriorly by the prevertebral fascia and posteriorly by the vertebral bodies and the posterior cervical musculature. It extends from the base of the skull to the coccyx.

Carotid space: The carotid space is located along the carotid sheath receiving contributions from the three deep cervical fascia, extending from the base of the skull to the mediastinum, which contains the internal carotid artery, internal jugular vein, cervical sympathetic chain and cranial nerves IX, X, XI, and XII.

Infrahyoid Spaces

Anterior visceral space: Located between the strap muscles and the esophagus, limited by the visceral division of the deep cervical fascia´s middle layer, it extends from the thyroid cartilage to the upper mediastinum, overlying the aortic arch and fibrous pericardium. It contains the thyroid gland, trachea and the anterior wall of the esophagus.

Etiology

DNI may be presented as a complication of several sources, although, dental origin is the most common in adults, and in many occasions, is the most aggressive. Other etiologies are: upper respiratory tract infections, intravenous drug abuse, and penetrating neck trauma. [1-5]. Infected sialoadenitis, sialolithiasis, paranasal sinuses, branchial sinuses or cysts, thyroglossal duct cysts and malignancies can appear as DNI and may be the first sign of disease. [5-11]

In the past, the most common source of DNI was pharyngitis, but throughout the years, there has been a relative increase in cases secondary to odontogenic infections, due to a growing number of patients with immune dysfunctions -as in HIV or diabetes mellitus-, low socioeconomic status and poor oral hygiene.

Pediatric DNI could represent a diagnostic challenge because their origin, location and microbial flora differs when compared to the adult population.

Staphylococcal species have a higher incidence in children and a greater propensity to infect peritonsillar and retropharyngeal spaces. [12-15]

In the past, retropharyngeal infections in adults were frequently related to tuberculosis, but now they are usually caused by trauma or foreign body ingestion.

Microbiology

It is well known that DNI, either in the pediatric population or adults, are polymicrobial. Only 5% may be identified as purely aerobic and 25% as purely anaerobic, although these microorganisms are difficult to assess. [17]

The fact polymicrobial cultures are grown from needle aspiration of deep neck abscesses, translates the oropharyngeal normal flora and odontogenic origin of most of these infections. The most frequently isolated aerobes are: *S viridans, Klebsiella pneumoniae*, and *S. aureus*; less frequently are: *Streptococcus pneumoniae*, *Streptococcus pyogenes*, Neisseria species, and *Haemophilus influenzae*. Common anaerobic isolates include *Peptostreptococcus, Bacteroides fragilis*, pigmented *Prevotella, Porphyromonas spp, Fusobacterium spp*, and *Eikenella corrodens.* [2, 13, 18-21] It is also well known that there is an increase in penicillin resistance due to β-lactamase production, which is released into the site of infection and protects nearby penicillin-sensitive species. [20] Group A streptococci represent the most common pathogen isolated in adults, although, *Prevotella* is the most common anaerobe. Several studies have demonstrated a higher incidence of *Staphylococcus aureus* in pediatric neck infections. [14, 16, 23, 24] In addition, methicillin resistant *S aureus* (MRSA), which is considered a nosocomial infection, has been diagnosed with increased prevalence as a community-acquired cause of DNI in: intravenous drug users, immunocompromised patients, infants, and young children, [13, 14, 22, 25-27] and in several geographical areas MRSA is an emerging pathogen in necrotizing fasciitis and descending mediastinitis [26, 28]. *K pneumoniae* is consistently the most common cause of DNI in uncontrolled diabetic patients. [1, 5, 29]

E corrodens is resistant to clindamycin and metronidazole and sensitive to penicillin and aminoglycosides. It is the most commonly isolated anaerobe in children and intravenous drug users. [13, 22] As mentioned before, DNI are polymicrobial either in adults and pediatrics, and β-lactamase organisms are becoming more and more frequent.

Diagnosis

In order to diagnose severe aggressive DNI infections, it is imperative to elaborate a meticulous history and physical examination. Physicians should assess important symptoms such as fever, pain, neck swelling, toothache, history of a dental procedure, intravenous drug use, upper respiratory tract infection, tonsillitis, sinusitis, trauma, skin abscess or cellulitis, with an adequate semiology for each symptom. It is very important to search all possible etiologies for DNI. Special attention should be made about symptoms suggesting airway compromise such as dysphagia, odynophagia, dyspnea, muffled voice, dysphonia, inability to handle secretions, and trismus, due to inflammation and irritation of nearby muscles of mastication. Patients with these symptoms can progress to a life-threatening compromise of the airway, so they represent a true surgical emergency. In children the presence of drooling, lymphadenopathy, fever, rhinorrhea, poor oral intake, and cough are important.

Physicians should also perform an efficient examination of the upper body. Inspection can reveal asymmetry of the face, head or neck. This may show areas of swelling, local erythema, an increase in the local temperature, and pustules. When these areas are palpated, consistency should be reported as firm or fluctuant, also changes in temperature and color, pain, fistulas or crepitus, which appears with gas-forming organisms. All triangles of the neck should be inspected and palpated in order to establish a topographical diagnosis. Moore´s sign is a simple maneuver that may reveal if the retropharyngeal space is occupied with fluid. With inspection of the oral cavity, physicians may notice elevation of the mouth´s floor with upward tongue displacement or purulent drainage through teeth or mucosae. Palate, tonsils and pharynx should be inspected and searched for asymmetries. Sometimes, flexible endoscopic exploration of the nose and pharynx may be useful when trismus is severe; this needs to be performed when oro-tracheal intubation is planned.

Infections involving the superficial cervical fascia may be evidenced as cellulitis in most cases, but they can also form abscesses, which must be drained.

A peritonsillar space infection originates from tonsillitis and it appears with a history of fever, pharyngodynia, dysphagia, muffled voice, trismus and cervical lymphadenopathy. Physical examination shows edema and tonsillar exudate, medial deviation of the lateral pharyngeal wall and uvula. It is always important to differentiate between an infection that has cellulitis or one that does require surgical drainage.

In the submandibular space, the roots of the second and third molars are posterior to the insertion of the mylohyoid muscle to the jaw, so dental infections can spread to the submandibular space, while infections originated in tooth roots that lie anterior to the muscle´s insertion will spread to the sublingual space, causing swelling, odinodysphagia, dysphagia or intense drooling which can progress to elevation of the mouth´s floor and tongue protrusion with upper airway obstruction, other possible origins of submandibular space infections are the ones found in secondary structures within it, such as sialadenitis, suppurative lymphadenitis, oral trauma, and upper respiratory infections.

Infections of the parapharyngeal space originate from propagation of neighboring structures such as pharyngeal or tonsillar infections, odontogenic infections, cervical lymphadenitis, otologic infections, Bezold`s abscess, and infections that involve the prestiloyd space present with: fever, chills, neck pain, trismus (by the inflammation of the medial pterygoid muscle) and displacement of the pharyngeal walls. Infections that involve the post-styloid space present with pain; and the presence of complications are more common, such as thrombosis of the internal jugular vein, carotid artery aneurysms, Horner´s syndrome and paralysis of cranial nerves IX, X, XI and XII.

Odontogenic infections originate from buccal space infections, appearing with: swelling, pain, hyperemia and trismus; these become evident when it spreads to the masseter muscle; systemic symptoms are rare.

Parotid space infections mostly result from obstruction of the parotid duct or from suppurated lymphadenitis, and occasionally from odontogenic origin; clinically, it presents with pain and acute inflammation, increased volume at the mandible´s angle, trismus, fever and malaise.

A retropharyngeal abscess is most common in the pediatric population, especially in children under 5 years old, usually due to infections of the respiratory tract, because the retropharyngeal lymph nodes receive drainage from the nose, sinuses and pharynx, it can also be secondary to trauma or infection of the parapharyngeal space. Clinically accompanied by cervical pain, swelling, fever, irritability, odinodysphagia, dysphagia, drooling, dyspnea and anorexia. In adult patients, nasal obstruction and snoring could be added.

Physical examination is found with a unilateral increase in volume of the posterior pharyngeal wall, the most feared complication of retropharyngeal abscesses is a mediastinitis.

Dangerous space infections are originated by contiguity from the preverterbal or retropharyngeal spaces, where the most common complication is a mediastinitis, because this space only contains loose areolar connective tissue that offers little resistance.

Prevertebral space infections originate secondary to: pharyngeal trauma, Pott`s abscess and infection of the retropharyngeal and danger spaces. Clinically manifested by an increase in volume of the posterior pharyngeal wall, with possible complications, such as osteomyelitis, spinal stability and hemiplegia.

Carotid space infections are due to: adjacent neck infections, direct inoculation by intravenous drug injections or iatrogenic causes, such as placement of central venous line, they have stiffness and swelling of the ipsilateral neck, fever, chills, ipsilateral Horner's syndrome or vocal cord palsy.

Visceral space infections are usually originated by traumatic perforations of the anterior esophageal wall, cervical trauma, or an infected thyroglossal cyst. They have cervical swelling, neck pain, pharyngodynia, dysphagia, dyspnea, dysphonia and crepitus. Medastinitis is a common complication after infections of this space (Figure 1).

Clinically, Ludwig’s angina is classically diagnosed by a rapidly spreading, firm, indurated cellulitis that originates intra-orally and bilaterally involves the sublingual and submaxilar spaces, but without abscess or lymphadenopathy, resulting in a rapidly progressing upper airway obstruction, most cases are of odontogenic origin; less common causes include peritonsillar or parapharyngeal abscesses, epiglottitis, and penetrating injuries to the floor of the mouth.

Swelling within the enclosed submandibular space displaces the tongue superiorly and posteriorly causing odynophagia, dysphagia, and drooling. Tongue protrusion can potentially culminate in rapid obstruction of the airway followed by asphyxiation if it is not urgently addressed.

It is also important to ask about comorbidities that may contribute to the progression of disease, as well as medical or surgical risk factors. Diabetes mellitus and other immunosuppressive –acquired or induced- diseases have been shown to contribute to a less favorable outcome for head, neck and other infections.

After a physical examination is performed, laboratory studies such as complete blood count, glucose, serum electrolytes, coagulation studies, liver and renal tests, HIV screening, blood cultures and isolations with needle aspiration for aerobic and anaerobic bacteria must be performed.

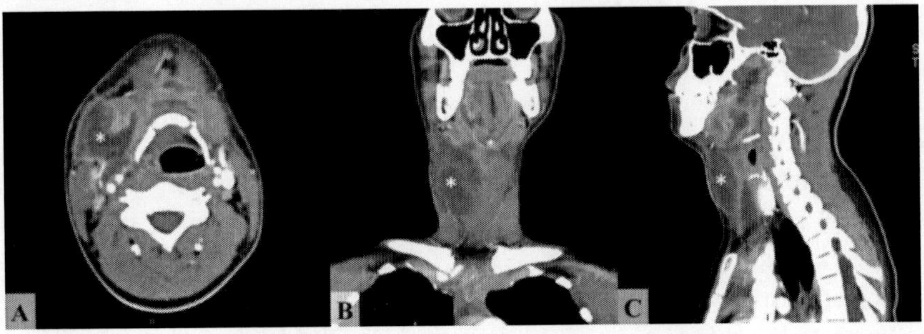

Figure 1. Axial (A), sagittal (B) and coronal (C) simple tomographic views of a patient who sustained an esophageal trauma showing subcutaneous and deep cervical emphysema with increased tissue density due to infection.

Diagnostic Imaging

After history taking and physical exploration have been performed, imaging studies should be ordered so that the surgeon can elaborate a more precise topographic diagnosis and an adequate medical and surgical treatment can be planned. Lateral x-rays of soft tissues of the neck are used to visualize thickening of the retropharyngeal, danger and/or prevertebral spaces; it is also useful to visualize thickening of the pre-epiglottic space. The presence of gas-forming bacteria or airway compromise may become evident in anterior-posterior and lateral.

The normal width of retropharyngeal space tissue in a lateral neck radiograph is 3.5 mm. in C_2, greater than 7 mm should be considered pathological; at C_6 level normal width should not exceed 14 mm in children and 22 mm in adults.

A chest X-ray is also essential in determining therapeutic planning, because it may indicate more severe complications, such as mediastinitis and pleural effusion.

Contrast-enhanced CT (CECT) is quite useful when characterizing deep neck lesions. Even if the presence of an abscess is suspected, CECT helps to elucidate if pus, cellulitis or none, occupy the spaces of the neck. It also helps physicians recognize potential complications, as well as planning for the most adequate surgical approach.

CECT is now days the current standard of care when managing a suspected DNI. [30] It is useful to identify impending airway complications before they present clinically. [25, 32] A cervical CECT extended to the thorax should be performed when neck swelling extends to the suprasternal notch or more because this may be indicative of a mediastinal involvement. [32] Serial CT or CECT scanning is useful in monitoring patients who have mediastinitis. [26] When a CECT is combined with careful examination, it has a 89% accuracy differentiating a drainable abscess from cellulitis. [31] CECT alone has an accuracy ranging from 63% [33] to 95% [34] in making this distinction. It has been suggested that a hypodensity greater than 2 mL in volume on CECT is more predictive of a deep neck abscess than the presence of a ring-enhancing lesion. [31]

CT is not 100% predictive when diagnosing DNI. The decision for surgical drainage should be made clinically, thus physical examination and CECT have been shown to be a critical component for the diagnosis of DNI (Figure 2).

Although, CECT helps to plan a surgical approach, Ultrasound is more accurate when differentiating cellulitis form abscess. [35] The advantages for ultrasound (US) are that it is portable, non-expensive, quick to perform, and it does not invade patients with radiation or intravenous contrast. Otherwise, ultrasound is difficult to interpret, it is operator-dependent, incapable to access deeper structures of the neck and does not help for surgical planning. [36] Therefore, US should be used as a supplement to CECT or MRI in cases when the presence of a deep neck abscess is unclear, and also to guide therapeutic needle aspiration when there is no airway compromise. [35] MRI is not used routinely, but it provides a better definition of soft tissue. [37] Magnetic resonance angiography is especially useful when vascular complications are suspected, such as internal jugular vein thrombophlebitis (IJVT), carotid aneurysms or rupture of neck vessels. [38]

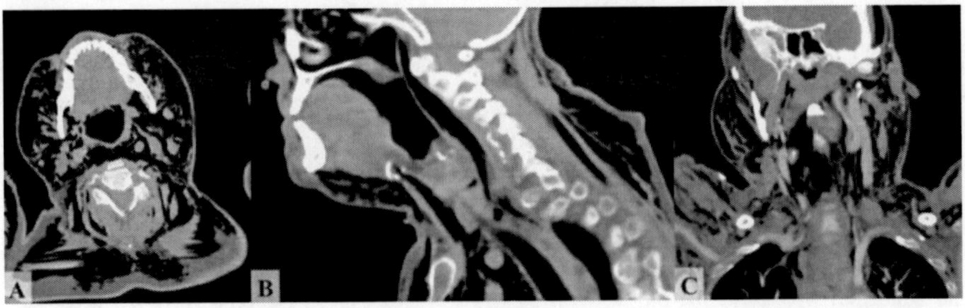

Figure 2. Axial (A), coronal (B) and sagittal (C) contrast-enhanced cervical tomographic views demonstrating a classical neck abscess (*asterisk*) with a potential for spread into the mediastinum.

Unfortunately, MRI is expensive and requires more time to perform, it may be necessary to sedate a child or a distressed patient, increasing the likelihood of airway compromise. [36]

Treatment

Aggressive monitoring and management of the airway are the most urgent and critical aspects of care, followed by appropriate antibiotic coverage and surgical drainage, when needed.

Empiric Antibiotic Coverage

Every patient who has a DNI should be treated with an initial empiric antibiotic therapy until culture and sensitivity results are available. Empirical treatment should be effective against aerobic and anaerobic bacteria that are commonly present in this kind of infections, the culture results with antibiotic testing allow to establish an appropriate treatment protocol.

Treatment could be started with empiric antibiotics such as cephalosporins like ceftriaxone, in addition to clindamycin, ensuring an adequate aerobic and anaerobic bacterial coverage, avoiding resistance to vancomycin or a penicillin combined with a β -lactamase inhibitor, amoxicillin with clavulanic acid, or a β-lactamase–resistant antibiotic (cefoxitin, cefuroxime, imipenem, or meropenem) with a drug that is highly effective against most anaerobes such as clindamycin or metronidazole is recommended for optimal empiric coverage. Vancomycin should be considered for empiric therapy in intravenous drug abusers at risk for infection with MRSA and in patients who have profound neutropenia or immune dysfunction. The addition of gentamicin for effective gram-negative coverage against *K. pneumoniae*, which is resistant to clindamycin, is highly recommended for diabetic patients.

Steroids

The use of steroids, along with antibiotic treatment in DNI management may reduce the need for surgical intervention by minimizing airway edema, inflammation and progression of cellulitis into an abscess, because of its strong anti-inflammatory effect, also helps in pain control, relieving dysphagia, and simplifying rehydration.

Airway Management

Acute airway obstruction is one of the most frequent and deadly complications. Careful airway monitoring is the first priority when treating any patient who has a DNI. Indications for aggressive airway management include signs of respiratory distress like: dyspnea, stridor, bronchospasm / impending airway compromise (noted on physical examination or diagnostic imaging), severe swelling within the pharynx, upward displacement of the tongue, and airway edema or compression by an abscess.

In advanced DNI cases, placing the patient in the supine position may precipitate a complete airway obstruction, which is important to consider when sedating a patient in the supine position, or sending them for an imaging study without first securing the airway.

Endotracheal intubation may be attempted before tracheotomy in most patients. However, it is often difficult due to a distorted anatomy of the airways, immobility of the soft tissues, or trismus that limit access to the mouth. Extreme care should be taken because of the risk of rupture and subsequent pus broncho-aspiration. In less severe infections, trismus may be controlled with the use of general anesthesia. However, in more advanced cases, general anesthesia is dangerous and can precipitate complete airway obstruction that could warrant an emergency tracheotomy.

The advantages of endotracheal intubation are fast airway control and avoidance of risks associated to a surgical procedure. Disadvantages include: airway edema, patient discomfort, a less secure airway, greater need for sedation / mechanical ventilation, and potential for a laryngo-tracheal stenosis. Unplanned extubation is the most common complication of an intubated patient.

Fiber optic nasotracheal intubation, when performed by experienced hands using topical anesthesia, is especially useful in patients who have severe trismus, granted airways are uncompromised.

Tracheotomy under local anesthesia is an indication for severe or impending airway obstruction when trismus or massive soft tissue edema precludes endotracheal intubation or when repeated attempts at intubation have failed. Separate incisions should be used for tracheotomy and drainage procedures of the anterior neck to avoid infectious spread into the mediastinum.

Surgical Indications

Surgical drainage is the first-line of treatment for patients in which the presence of an abscess within deep neck spaces is suspected. [32, 38, 39] Recent studies, however, suggest that, in several cases and in which there is no evidence of complications, DNI may be treated only with antibiotics. It has been established that comorbidities such as uncontrolled diabetes, may be treated with insulin simultaneously with antibiotic therapy, improving their immune system. Conservative treatment does not increase mortality or length of hospitalization in DNI. [40] In patients with cellulitis, the use of steroids in combination with antibiotic treatment reduces the need for surgical intervention by minimizing airway / mucosa edema, inflammation, and progression of cellulitis into an abscess. [29, 40] Oh *et al.* [41] found that 55.9% of 34 parapharyngeal space abscesses responded well to conservative medical management. When encountered with an immunocompromised patient or anyone at risk of infection with atypical or nosocomial bacteria, aspiration and culture are quite necessary. [35]

As mentioned, surgical intervention is the mainstay of treatment for more complicated or severe DNI cases. Indications for surgery include: airway compromise, critical condition, septicemia, complications, descending infection, diabetes mellitus, or no clinical improvement within 48 hours of initial parenteral antibiotic treatment. [1, 35, 37] In our experience, abscesses greater than 3 cm that involve more than two spaces or involve the prevertebral, anterior visceral, or carotid spaces, should be surgically drained.

Surgical Technique

Surgical drainage can be performed in several ways, including a simple intra- or extra-oral incision and drainage for superficial abscesses, a more extensive external cervical approach for deeper and more complicated infections, and minimally invasive techniques such as image-guided needle aspiration and indwelling catheter placement. Abscesses that are small and unilocular may respond well to needle aspiration, whereas larger and multilocular abscesses usually require surgical drainage. [35] Regardless of the approach, surgical specimen should be sent for gram stain and cultures, as soon as the abscess cavity is entered. [37]

Surgical access of the parapharyngeal space has traditionally been by way of an external cervical approach, with an incision along the border of the sternocleidomastoid muscle to gain adequate exposure and avoid injuring carotid sheath contents.

The surgical approach for the exposure and drainage of the masticator space depends on the abscess´ location in relation to the mandible. An intraoral approach at the retromolar trigone is appropriate for draining abscesses medial to the ramus of the mandible, and an extra-oral approach along the inferior border of the mandible is used for draining abscesses lateral to the mandibular ramus. An incision through the temporalis fascia along the hairline is necessary to drain abscesses that spread superiorly and surround the temporalis muscle within the temporal space.

An external, parotidectomy-like approach is used to drain a parotid space abscess, and blunt dissection, either superior or inferior to the posterior belly of the digastric muscle, allows concurrent drainage of the parapharyngeal space when it is involved.

The approach for draining a retropharyngeal abscess depends in its location, if it's in the nasopharynx, a guided puncture is recommended; if it's at the level of the oropharynx, a trans-oral drainage by a vertical incision in the posterior and lateral pharyngeal wall is indicated; if the abscess is in the hypopharynx, an external cervical approach should be performed, with a horizontal incision at the level of the hyoid, sternocleidomastoid muscle and retracting laterally the neuro-vascular bundle by blunt dissection.

Wide exposure of the infected tissue is important, as is debridement of any necrotic tissue present. Wounds requiring extensive debridement should be left open and packed with antimicrobial dressings to allow for frequent inspection, this allows better tissue oxygenation, reducing anaerobic flora. In our experience, it is preferred to inspect and debride twice a day while the wound remains open and pathologic fluids are obtained. Wounds with less necrosis can be closed at surgery with active suction or Penrose drainages. In cases that involve descending infections, cervical drainage is sufficient as long as the infection remains above the carina; transthoracic drainage is necessary when infection spreads below the carina. [37] Minimally invasive techniques have been used more recently for well-defined, unilocular abscesses in patients who do not have airway compromise. Ultrasound guidance may be appropriate for locating and draining abscesses accessible through the skin, and CT guidance is helpful when attempting needle aspiration of a deep, difficult to access fluid collection. Needle aspiration and catheter placement offer the advantages of a small point of entry, faster healing time, little or no scar formation, and less risk of contaminating the surrounding deep neck spaces while draining pus.

Post-Operative Treatment

After medical and surgical treatments have resolved the infectious process, the wound should be stitched, if not possible, it is left open and it should close by second intention. When the patient is discharged, daily wound care is recommended at home and during visits (every 5 days) at the Outpatient Clinic, surgical wound status should be followed with stitch removal after 7 days, closely monitoring for seroma formation or reactivation.

If the source was secondary to odontogenic infection, the patient should be sent to de dentist for teeth evaluation and removal, if necessary. Continued oral antibiotic treatment is recommended until the wound is completely closed.

Complications

Mediastinal Extension

Acute mediastinitis is a severe infection of the connective tissue that fills the mediastinal space surrounding middle thoracic organs, which is caused by downward spread of DNI.

There are several routes for infection from the neck to mediastinum. The most important route for a descending infection is the retropharyngeal, prevertebral, danger, carotid and visceral space.

The higher risk for developing a complicated course of DNI with worse prognosis is especially in older patients with comorbidities, such as cardiovascular and pulmonary diseases.

Internal Jugular Vein Thrombophlebitis

It is the result of an infectious extension into the carotid space. Pathognomonic findings include: swelling and tenderness at the angle of the jaw and along the sternocleidomastoid muscle, signs of sepsis (spiking fevers, chills) and evidence of pulmonary emboli. The mechanism of vascular thrombosis is attributed to Virchow's triad, which is: endothelial damage, hypercoagulability, and blood flow abnormalities; all these initiate a thrombotic process. IJVT may be diagnosed using high-resolution ultrasound, CECT, or MRI. When a thrombus progresses or a septic emboli is present, treatment involves prolonged tailored antimicrobial therapy, and anticoagulation for 3 months; most cases resolve and do not require surgical ligation and resection of the internal jugular vein.

Carotid Artery Aneurysm

A carotid artery aneurysm may present with a pulsatile neck mass that often results in four cardinal signs: Recurrent sentinel hemorrhages from the pharynx or ear, protracted clinical course (7–14 days), hematoma of the surrounding tissues, hemodynamic collapse. Early recognition and surgical intervention to gain proximal control of the common carotid artery is essential, because a more distal ligation may be impossible. Interventional radiologic procedures such as endovascular stenting or vessel occlusion are also an option in less urgent cases.

Necrotizing Cervical Fasciitis

This is a fulminant infection that spreads along fascial planes and causes necrosis of connective tissues. Patients who have necrotizing fasciitis are acutely ill with high fevers and damage to the skin, showing superficial necrosis that may be tender, edematous, and erythematous, with indistinct transition with normal skin underneath it. Soft tissue crepitation due to infection with gas-producing organisms may be present, and, in more advanced cases, the skin becomes pale, anesthetic, and dusky, with blistering and sloughing. The pathogens involved are usually polymicrobial and odontogenic, and they include *S pyogenes*, *Clostridium perfringens* , and mixed aerobes and anaerobes. MRSA has recently been recognized as an important cause. Managing necrotizing fasciitis should be in an ICU and involves parenteral antibiotics along with early and frequent surgical debridement of any devitalized tissue. The wound should be left open and packed with antimicrobial dressings until the infection has subsided. Hyperbaric oxygen is useful as an adjunctive treatment in hemodynamically stable patients. The condition is often accompanied by mediastinitis and sepsis, which increase the risk of mortality, justifying the use of this therapy in high risk patients.

Conclusion

Deep neck infections today is a disease that has had a significant decrease in incidence but its complications have a high mortality rate, so it is important to make an accurate diagnosis and timely treatment so to avoid extension and unfortunate aoutcomes such as descending necrotizing mediastinits.

References

[1] Huang T. T., LIU T. C., Chen P. R., Tseng F. Y., Yeh T. H., Chen Y. S. Deep neck infection: analysis ok 185 cases. *Head Neck* 2004; 26(10): 854-860.

[2] Har-El G., Aroesty J. H., Shana A., Lucente F. E. Changing trends in deep neck abscess: a retrospective study of 110 patients. *Oral Surg Oral Med Oral Pathol* 1994;77(5):1051-1054.

[3] Parhiscar A., Har-El G., Deep neck abscess: a retrospective review of 210 cases. *Ann Otol Rhinol Laryngol.*, 2001; 110(11):1051-1054.

[4] Sethi D. S., Stanley R. E. Deep neck abscesses-changing trends. *J Laryngol Otol* 1994;108(2):138-143.

[5] Lee J. K., Kim H. D., Lim S. C. Predisponing factors of complicated deep neck infections: an analysis of 158 cases. *Yonsei Med J* 2007; 48(1): 55-62.

[6] Brook I. Microbiology and management of peritonsillar, retropharyngeal, and parapharyngeal abscesses. *J Oral Maxilofac Surg* 2004; 62(12):1545-1550.

[7] Brook I. Microbiology and management of infected solid tumours. *Eur J. Cancer Care* 2007; 16(1):12-16.

[8] Nusbaum A. O., Som P. M., Rothschild M. A., Shugar J. M. Recurrence of a deep neck infection: a clinical indication of an underlying congenital lesión. *Arch Otolaryngol Head Neck Surg* 1999;125(12): 1279-1282.

[9] Ostlie D. J., Burjonrappa S. C., Snyder C. L., Watts J., Murphy J. P., Gittes G. K., Andrews W. A., Sharp R. J., Holcomb G. W. 3rd. Thyroglossal duct infections and surgical outcomes. *J Pediatr Surg* 2004;39(3):396-399.

[10] Park S. W., Han M. H., Sung M. H., Kim I. O., Kim K. H., Chang K. H., Han M. C. Neck infection associated with pyriform sinus fistula: imaging findings. *AJNR Am J Neuroradiol* 2000; 21(5):817-822.

[11] Wang C. P., Ko J. Y., Lou P. J. Deep neck infection as the main initial presentation of primary head and neck cáncer. *J Laryngol Otol* 2006; 120(4): 305-309.

[12] Choi S. S., Vezina L. G., Grundfast K. M. Relative incidence and alternative approaches for surgical drainage of different types of deep neck abscesses in children. *Arch Otolaryngol Head Neck Surg* 1997; 123(12): 1275-1275.

[13] Coticcia J. M., Getnick G. S., Yun R. D., Arnold J. E. Age-, site-, and time-specific differences in pediatric deep neck abscesses. *Arch Otolaryngol Head Neck Surg* 2004;130(2):201-207.

[14] Tan P. M., Chang L. Y., Huang Y. C., Chiu C. H., Wang C. R., Lin T. Y. Deep neck infections in children. *J Microbiol Infect* 2001; 34(4): 287-292.

[15] Ungkanont K., Yellon R. F., Weissman J. L., Casselbrant M. L., González-Valdepeña H., Bluestone C. D. Head and neck space infections in infants and children. *Otolaryngol Head Neck Surg* 1995; 112(3): 375-382.

[16] Marioni G., Castegnaro E., Steffieri C., Rinaldi R., Giacomelli L., Boninsegna M., Bertolin A., Staffieri A. Deep neck infection in elderly patients: a single institution experience (200-2004). *Aging Clin Exp Res* 2006;18(2):127-132.

[17] Brook I. Microbiology and principles of antimicrobial therapy for head and neck infections. *Infect Dis Clin North Am* 2007; 21(2) 355-391.

[18] Weed H. G., Forest L. A. Deep neck infection. In: Cummings C. W., Flint P. W., Harker L. A., et al, editors. Otolaryngology: head and neck surgery, vol. 3. 4th edition. Philadelphia: Elsevier Mosby; 2005. p. 2515–2524.

[19] Parhiscar A., Har-El G. Deep neck abscess: a retrospective review of 210 cases. *Ann Otol Rhinol Laryngol* 2001;110(11):1051–1054.

[20] Brook I. Anaerobic bacteria in upper respiratory tract and other head and neck infections. *Ann Otol Rhinol Laryngol* 2002;111:430–40.

[21] Thompson J., Cohen S., Reddix P. Retropharyngeal abscess in children: a retrospective and historical analysis. *Laryngoscope* 1988;98(6):589–592.

[22] Lee K., Tami T., Echavez M., Wildes T. O. Deep neck infections in patients at risk for acquired immunodeficiency syndrome. *Laryngoscope* 1990;100(9):915–919.

[23] Chen M. K., Wen Y. S., Chang C. C., Lee H. S., Huang M. T., Hsiao H. C. Deep neck infection in diabetes patients. *Am J Otolaryngol* 2000; 21(3):169-173.

[24] Huang T. T., Tseng F. Y., Liu T. C., Hsu C. J., Chen Y. S. Deep neck infection in diabetic patients: comparison of clinical picture and outcomes with nondiabetic patients. *Otolaryngol Head Neck Surg* 2005; 132(2):355-391.

[25] Cmejrek R., Coticchia J., Arnold J. Presentation, diagnosis, and management of deep-neck abscesses in infants. *Arch Otolaryngol Head Neck Surg* 2002;128(12):1361–1364.

[26] Naidu S., Donepudi S., Stocks R., Buckingham S. C., Thompson J. W. Methicillin-resistant Staphylococcus aureus as a pathogen in deep neck abscesses: a pediatric case series. *Int J Pediatr Otorhinolaryngol* 2005; 69(10):1367–1371.

[27] Sato K., Izumi T., Toshima M., Nagai T., Muroi K., Komatsu N., Ozawa K. Retropharyngeal abscess due to methicillin-resistant Staphylococcus aureus in a case of acute myeloid leukemia. *Intern Med* 2005;44(4): 346–349.

[28] Miller L., Perdreau-Remington F., Rieg G., Mehdi S., Perlroth J., Bayer A. S., Tang A. W., Phung T. O., Spellberg B. Necrotizing fasciitis caused by community associated methicillin-resistant Staphylococcus aureus in Los Angeles. *N Engl J Med* 2005;352(14):1445–1453.

[29] Wang L., Kuo W., Tsai S., Huang K. J. Characterizations of life-threatening deep cervical space infections: a review of one hundred ninety-six cases. *Am J Otolaryngol* 2003; 24(2):111–117.

[30] Boscolo-Rizzo P., Marchiori C., Zanetti F., Vaglia A., Da Mosto M. C. Conservative management of deep neck abscesses in adults: the importance of CECT findings. *Otolaryngol Head Neck Surg* 2006; 135(6): 894–899.

[31] Miller W., Furst I., Sandor G., Keller M. A. A prospective, blinded comparison of clinical examination and computed tomography in deep neck infections. *Laryngoscope* 1999;109(11):1873–1879.

[32] Crespo A., Chone C., Fonseca A., Montenegro M. C., Pereira R., Milani J. A. Clinical versus computed tomography evaluation in the diagnosis and management of deep neck infection. *Sao Paulo Med J* 2004; 122(6): 259–263.

[33] Vural C., Gungor A., Comerci S. Accuracy of computerized tomography in deep neck infections in the pediatric population. *Am J Otolaryngol* 2003; 24(3):143–148.

[34] Nagy M., Pizzuto M., Backstrom J., Brodsky L. Deep neck infections in children: a new approach to diagnosis and treatment. *Laryngoscope* 1997;107(12):1627–1634.

[35] Yellon R. F. Head and neck space infections. In: Bluestone C. D., Casselbrant M. L., Stool S. E., editors. Pediatric otolaryngology, vol. 2. 4th edition. Philadelphia: Saunders; 2003. p. 1681–1701.

[36] Smith J., Hsu J., Chang J. Predicting deep neck space abscess using computed tomography. *Am J Otolaryngol* 2006;27(4):244–247.

[37] Weed H. G., Forest L. A. Deep neck infection. In: Cummings C. W., Flint P. W., Harker L. A., et al, editors. Otolaryngology: head and neck surgery, vol. 3. 4th edition. Philadelphia: Elsevier Mosby; 2005. p. 2515–2524.

[38] Gidley P., Ghorayeb B., Stiernberg C. Contemporary management of deep neck space infections. *Otolaryngol Head Neck Surg* 1997;116(1): 16–22.

[39] Ridder G., Technau-Ihling K., Sander A., Boedeker C. C. Spectrum and management of deep neck space infections: an 8-year experience of 234 cases. *Otolaryngol Head Neck Surg* 2005;133(5):709–714.

[40] Mayor G., Millan J., Martinez-Vidal A. Is conservative treatment of deep neck space infections appropriate? *Head Neck* 2001;23(2):126–133.

[41] Oh J., Kim Y., Kim C. Parapharyngeal abscess: comprehensive management protocol. *ORL J Otorhinolaryngol Relat Spec* 2007;69(1): 37–42.

[42] Celakovsky P., Kalafert D., Tucek L., Mejzlik J., Kotulek M., Vrbacky A., Matousek P., Stanikova L., Hoskova T., Pasz A. Deep neck infections: risk factors for mediastinal extension, *Eur Arch Otorhinolaryngol* 2014;271(6):1679-1683.

[43] Hasegawa J., Hidaka H., Tateda M., Kudo T., Sagai S., Miyazaki M., Katagiri K., Nakanome A., Ishida E., Ozawa D., Kobayashi T. (2011) An analysis of clinical risk factors of deep neck infection. *Auris Nasus Larynx* 2011;38(1):101–107.

In: Mediastinal Infections
Editor: Walid Leonardo Dajer-Fadel
ISBN: 978-1-63463-369-7

Chapter 3

Descending Necrotizing Mediastinitis

***W. L. Dajer-Fadel*[1]* *and C. Ibarra-Pérez*[2]**
[1] Cardiothoracic Surgery Department, General Hospital of Mexico "Dr. Eduardo Liceaga", Mexico City, Mexico
[2] National Academy of Medicine, Mexico City, Mexico

Abstract

Descending necrotizing mediastinitis (DNM) is one of the most dreadful infections in medicine, originated from a superior site above the thoracic cavity that eventually extends through the cervical spaces and fascia into one of the pathways of descent, opening its way into the mediastinum causing an overwhelming septic process that left untouched, could cause the patient´s death. There are now strict diagnostic criteria that the physician needs to search for when treating this rare group of patients to achieve the best possible outcome. The chapter will discuss how these present to the ER and what are the adequate processes that have to be set in motion to save their lives. All the information presented will be correlated to the best up to date available evidence and the authors´ institutional results where the largest series of patients has been published. It is of the utmost importance that this disease is identified in a timely fashion so that emergent surgical drainage and lavage of the

* Correspondence to: Walid Leonardo Dajer-Fadel, E-mail Address: drdajer@gmail.com.

mediastinal spaces are performed, followed with resuscitation at an Intensive Respiratory Care Unit, being vigilant of the patient´s metabolic / immunologic response and a watchful eye to possible post-operative complications that may arise so they could be treated in the earliest manner.

Introduction

Historically DNM has been a major disease accounting for almost 100% mortality before the pre-antibiotic era with partial decline in contemporary times. [1] Even with the best technology available, it still worries thoracic surgeons around the world due to its high death rate. As we will see in the chapter, the majority of patients suffer from some kind of immunosuppression that complicates healing and resolution of their septic process, surgery is still the first line of treatment against this dreadful disease, it has always been hypothesized that the earlier it is diagnosed and treated the better the outcome. In earlier years diagnosis was made from a suspicion based in the clinical and para-clinical data summoned by a simple chest X-ray that now we know it has a low sensitivity and specificity, this improved in later years thanks to computed tomography imaging for earlier diagnosis; surgical techniques have varied over time with postero-lateral thoracotomies, sternotomies, subxifoid or cervical incisions, but as time goes by, video-assisted thoracic surgery (VATS) is becoming the standard of care. Also, postoperative treatment is very important at the Intensive Respiratory Care Unit (IRCU). In a whole, to achieve the best results for these patients, it is imperative that care must be done by a multidisciplinary team of experts that treat a relative high volume of cases, under these circumstances, higher rates of success are reached. In this chapter we will discuss every aspect of diagnosis, treatment and outcomes, offering a treatment algorithm for future reference.

Etiology

The origin of cervical infections are as follows: odontogenic (Ludwig´s angina) 45%, retropharyngeal 25%, cervical abscesses 11.7%, esophageal perforation (EP) 8.3% and other 10% (Figures 1 & 2). [2] These sites are in direct correlation to the cervical spaces and fascia. Ludwig´s angina is an infection of the second and third molars that extends to the tooth´s root reaching the submandibular space, if the abscess is not controlled at this point, its prone to invade contiguous spaces such as the masseter or parapharyngeal which eventually reach the retropharyngeal and retroesophageal spaces until it spreads to the mediastinum, almost invariably when this space is affected the infection spreads beyond the tracheal carina.

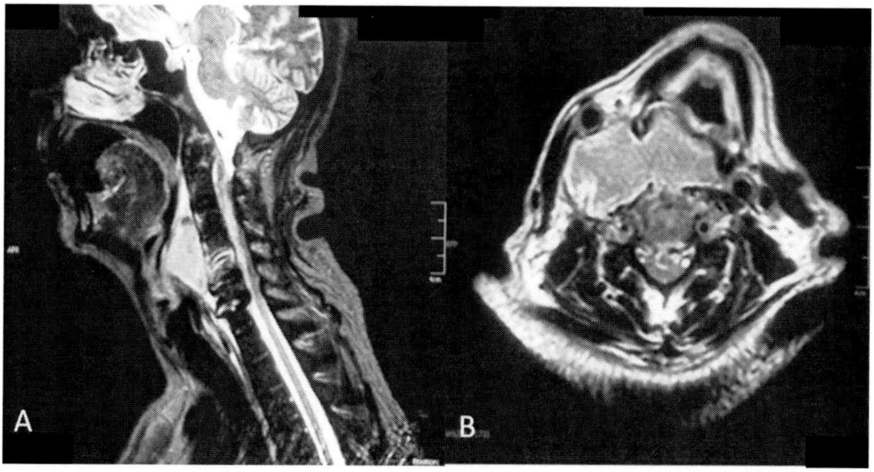

Figure 1. (A) Sagittal T2-weightned magnetic resonance image demonstrating an abscess with medullary compression and cervical spondylolisthesis. (B) Axial T2-weightned image showing it with direct vertebral body invasion and inflammation. (Reproduced with permission).

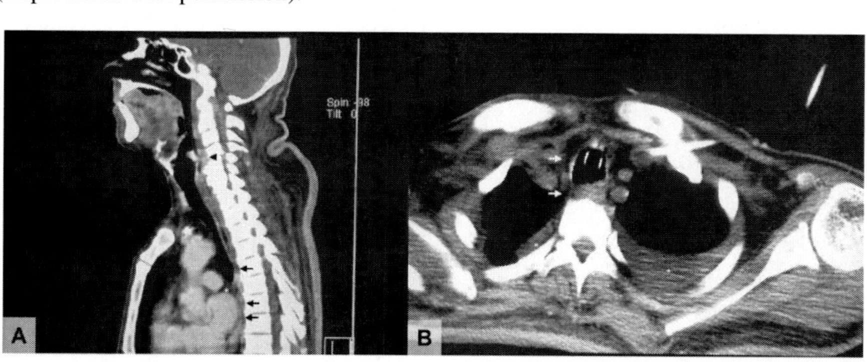

Figure 2. Same patient as figure 1 with a (A) computed tomography in sagittal view demonstrating heterogeneity of adipose tissue of the posterior mediastinum (asterisk) and dissection of the retroesophageal space (arrows) secondary to a cervical infection (arrowhead). (B) Axial view of upper mediastinum with dissection of the anterior mediastinum (arrows) and bilateral pleural effusion (asterisks). (Reproduced with permission).

Therefore these patients have a clinical picture that comprises swelling of the neck, odynophagia, fever and trismus, associated with a low socio-cultural status. [3] It is of the outmost importance to prioritize airway management, due to a potential complication such as asphyxia. [4] Peritonsillar and cervical infections involve an inflammatory response in the contiguous tissues invading until it reaches the spaces in similar fashion.

Some authors don´t consider EP as an etiological factor for DNM, however when its proximal portion has a lesion and the criteria are met, there is no reason to discard it as a precursor of DNM. The most common cause for this lethal disease is iatrogenic (in 70% of the cases) due to endoscopic procedures (trans-esophagic ultrasonography, pneumatic dilation, endo-prothesis and failed oro-tracheal intubations) or just by the elevated number of endoscopies performed these days; followed by spontaneous rupture (Borhaave´s syndrome) in 15% of cases, typically 2-6 cm above the hiatus, foreign bodies, trauma (by a bullet wound or a knife) and even thoracic surgery procedures (mediastinoscopy, lymphadenectomy, myotomy, funduplicature, chest tubes that erode the esophagus due to proximity); delay in the treatment of this condition occurs in more than 50% of the cases. [5-7] This could be due to rupture during a procedure that went unseen or also related to a small lesion making it clinically evident many hours after the event. Risk factors for EP are: a) performing esophagoscopy without sufficient sedation, b) study done by an unexperienced operator, c) inadequate or insufficient material, d) biopsing lymph nodes without direct visualization and e) not collapsing the balloon of the oro-tracheal cannula when passing the endoscope.

Other rare causes of DNM have been described, such as varicella infection, spinal cord abscess (Figures 1 & 2), sterno-clavicular joint osteomyelitis (Figures 3 & 4), even skin infections which produce a rapidly evolving fasciitis that utimatelly invades deeper tissue planes, among others. [8-11] As long as diagnostic criteria are met, no matter how rare the cause of DNM, it should always be treated with the respect it deserves.

The most frequent microorganisms vary in a great deal from *Streptococcus β-haemolyticus*, (8.3 – 71.5%), *Pseudomonas aeruginosa* (26.7%), *Acinetobacter baumanii* (16.7%), depending from one author to another; it usually is a polymicrobial infection (in 44.4% of the cases) and many times with flora from the oral cavity. It is important to note that aerobic microorganisms cause thrombosis of small arteries favoring the growth of anaerobic flora. [1,12]

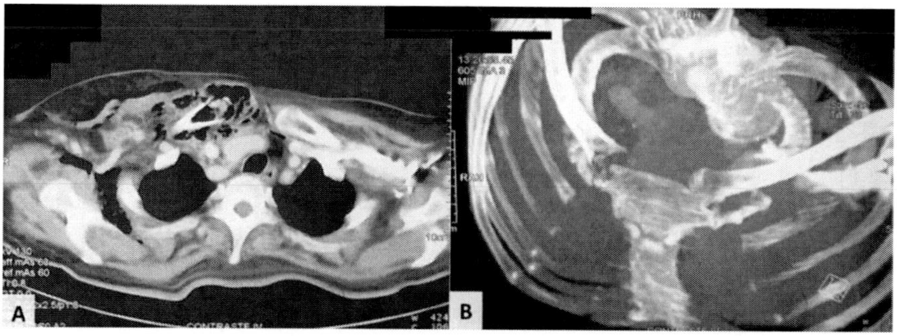

Figure 3. (A) Contrast-enhanced chest tomographic scan showing destruction of the sternoclavicular joint and surrounding tissues, with extension into the superior mediastinum. (B) Tomographic reconstruction of the thoracic outlet revealing the extent of bone damage. (Reproduced with permission).

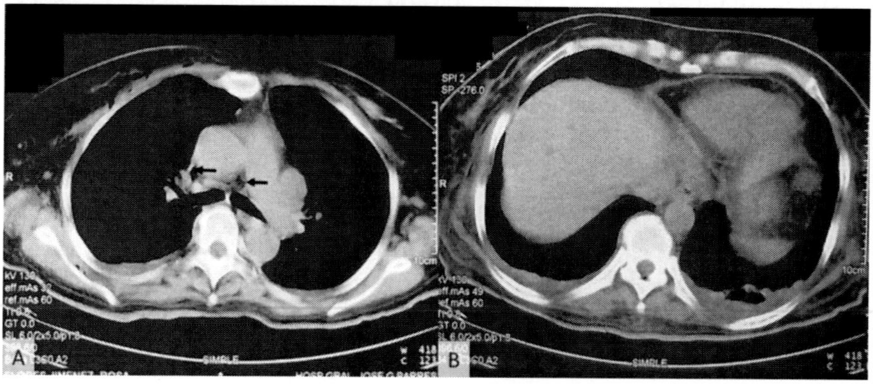

Figure 4. Same patient as figure 3 with an (A) axial tomographic view demonstrating peritracheal gas (arrows). (B) Lower view of the same scan, showing bilateral pleural effusions. (Reproduced with permission).

Risk Factors Associated to Descending Necrotizing Mediastinitis

Patients that suffer from DNM usually arrive to the ER with multiple comorbidities (46.7%), such as type 2 diabetes mellitus (33.3%), osteo-articular rheumatic diseases (8.3%), hypertension (6.7%), immunosuppression (3.3%) and other (13.3%), 15% of the time they have more than one, this is the reason why searching for risk factors that influence death with statistical significance is so important, few publications have looked into this. According to a study of 60 patients with DNM, 66.5% of patients with comorbidities died compared to 35.9% of the ones that did not (p=<0.05) especially diabetic patients (20% *vs.* 57%), age ≥50 years-old (mean of 36.4 *vs.* 49.9), and complications (61.5% *vs.*100%); it may not be a risk factor but the mean number of survival days for the deceased was five compared to the length of stay at the hospital for survivors of 22.5 days. Other authors concluded that only septic shock is a risk factor for mortality. Curiously time from symptoms to arrival at the ER and from seeking medical attention until operated were analyzed but no significant threshold in hours or days was found.[2] Deu-Martín *et al.* [13] in a study of 43 patients found that a diagnostic period from 1996-2000 compared to modern times made a difference in mortality, however many reports still have high mortality rates in recent years; in their bivariate analysis they also found that diabetes mellitus, comorbidities, number of surgeries, left lateral thoracotomy, postoperative morbidity (complications) and septic shock were significant for increased mortality. Table 1 synthesizes the risk factors for mortality.

Table 1. Risk factors for mortality in DNM

Author	Significant risk factors
Dajer-Fadel et al.[2]	Comorbidities (diabetes mellitus) Age above 50 years-old Complications
Deu-Martin et al.[13]	Diagnosis period 1996-2000 Diabetes mellitus Comorbidity Number of surgeries Left lateral surgery Postoperative morbidity Septic shock

Diagnosis

The most important pathways for descent in DNM are the pre-tracheal and pre-vertebral fascia, which are ultimately communicated to the pre-vascular, visceral and retrovisceral zones. [14] When a cervical infection is imminent it can extend to any of the mediastinal compartments being the retrovisceral zone the most commonly affected. Type 2 diabetes mellitus (42%) is the most common comorbidity associated with these patients followed by systemic arterial hypertension (12%) and immunosupresion (8%) of any kind. [15] According to Estrera *et al.*[16] to diagnose DNM the following criteria are required: a) clinical manifestations of an acute oropharyngeal infection; b) radiological findings of mediastinitis; c) intra-operative (Figure 5) or post-mortem evidence of necrotizing mediastinitis; and d) a direct correlation between the oropharyngeal process and development of DNM. These have all to be considered during disgnostic work up, however physicians have to always get into the context of the patient, such as how and when the original infection started, review his or her blood work in the lookout for leukocytosis or elevation of acute phase reactants. It is the authors' point of view that when a diagnostic suspicion is imminent, the patient has to invariably undergo surgery and if the criteria are not fulfilled after the procedure, it is still acceptable, due to the fact that when septic shock kicks in, there is a very minute chance for survival.

The standard of care for a preoperative diagnosis is a contrast-enhanced CT which allows identification of both, the source of infection and the route of spread. Findings include fluid collection within the mediastinum, heterogeneity of the mediastinal adipose tissue, localized gas within the mediastinum, pericardial or pleural effusions, empyema, and / or pneumopericardium (Figure 6), more on radiological diagnosis and anatomical correlation will be discussed in the next chapters. [17]

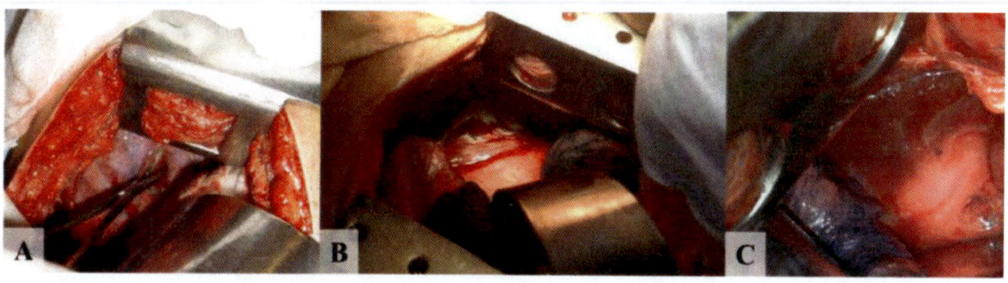

Figure 5. Presence of purulent exudate of the retrovisceral (A), visceral (B) and prevascular (C) zones during surgery.

Classification

As all diseases, it is always useful to classify them, generally based on their severity; this process aids in making decisions for treatment protocols or as prognostic information demonstrated by survival studies. Endo *et al.*[18] first described a classification based on tomographic evidence of tissue involvement, defined as: type I which refers to diffusion of infection above the tracheal carina, type IIA reaches beyond the tracheal carina involving the anterior mediastinum, and Type IIB which occupies the same area as the previous but also the posterior mediastinum (Figure 7).

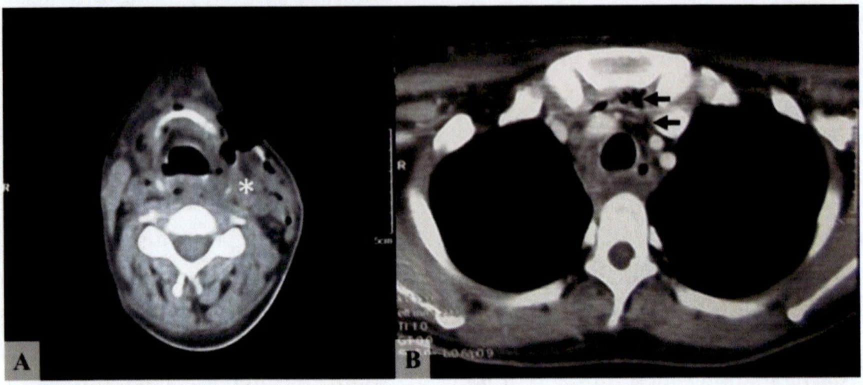

Figure 6. Axial (A) cervical tomographic view with threatening abscess (asterisk) that dissected until it reached the mediastinum (B), where gas collection and heterogeneity of the anterior mediastinal adipose tissue is seen (arrows).

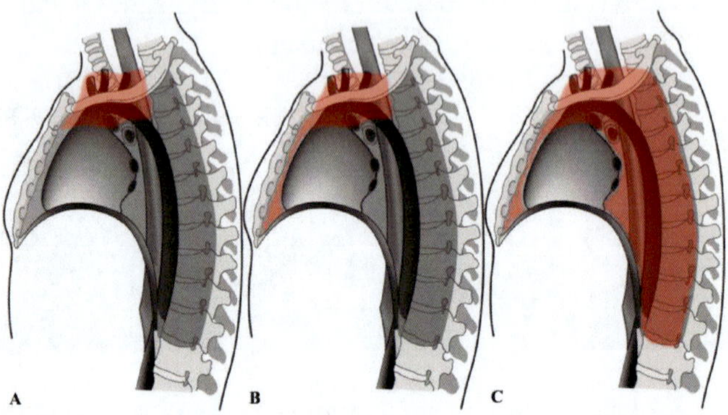

Figure 7. Schematic representation of Endo´s classification for spread of disease in DNM: (A) type I, (B) type IIA, (C) type IIB.

The authors believe this classification to be impractical since there is no clear difference (prognostic and treatment wise) between type IIA and type IIB, also, in his work, his group based it upon four patients only. Recently a modification was proposed dividing it only in superior DNM (above tracheal carina) and inferior DNM (when extension showed below the tracheal carina) based on 100 patients (Figure 8), where there was a significance in mortality between both groups, being lower for the superior type (10.3% *vs.* 36.6%) with patients being operated just by a cervicotomy, while in the inferior type they were approached through a cervicotomy plus a right thoracotomy; the authors concluded that inferior DNM represented an important risk factor for mortality, and that the inferior type also carries a greater burden on the patient`s immunologic and systemic inflammatory response. [15]

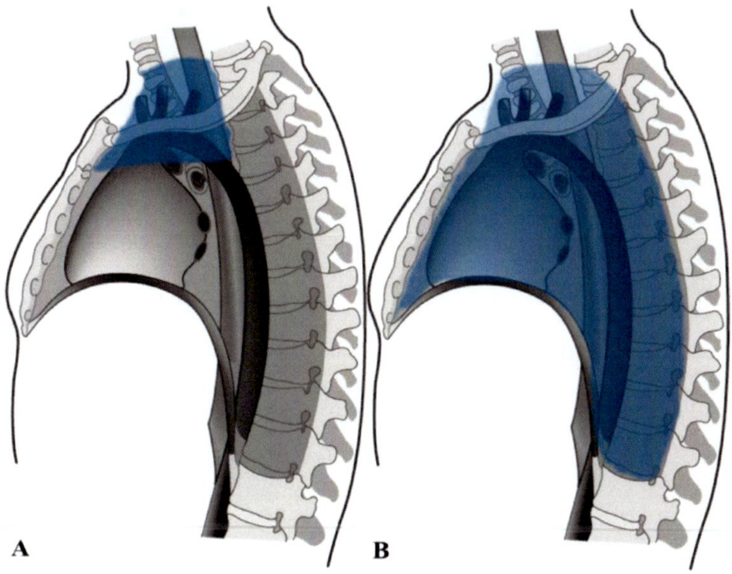

Figure 8. Schematic representation of the authors´ simplified version of DNM classification: (A) superior DNM, (B) inferior DNM.

Severity Scoring

The Thoracic Surgery Scoring System (Thoracoscore) is a mortality predictor score for hospitalized patients after a general thoracic surgery is performed. It was originally calculated based on 15 183 patients in whom a thoracic procedure was performed from 59 institutions. It is calculated before the intervention. [19,20] Thoracoscore has been validated in the literature with excellent results. [21] However, the authors have used this system in patients with DNM without success validating it. [2]

SAPS3, is a scoring system based on physiological abnormalities that has proved success grading the severity of a disease in patients with "critical" illnesses. [22] It utilizes the information of the first day of stay at the ICU to calculate the probability of death. [23] The authors believe this is the most accurate from of scoring based on its background however no studies have been performed analyzing it for DNM.

Treatment

When patients arrive at the ER with cervical discomfort or swelling and imaging studies that are suspicious for DNM, medical treatment should be started with antibiotics (ceftriaxone and clindamyacin); immediately the OR should be prepared to undergo cervical and/or mediastinal lavage and drainage of all spaces so no collections are left out. This procedure is performed in some centers by otorrhynolaringologists and thoracic surgeons; or only by the latter with acceptable results from both groups. Currently there is no study that compares results made by one group or another. Details on the technique will be discussed in the following chapters. After successful mediastinal drainage, the patient has to continue treatment –ideally- at a Respiratory Intensive Care Unit, for continued wound care, mostly of the cervicotomy, since sometimes this incision is left open for subsequent lavage and drainage at the ICU; and when adequate evolution is seen, a second or third intention wound closure is planned. For the thoracic part, follow up daily chest x-rays are taken to evaluate the thoracic cavity, ideally another CT scan should be performed 48 – 72 hours after the intervention to re-evaluate fluid collections and appropriate drainage of the mediastinal spaces and fascia. It is very important to send samples for microbial culturing to tailor antibiotic treatment during the postoperative period, always remember that in some occasion no growth is going to be present in DNM. Rehabilitation is a very important aspect to consider during treatment, it is most important that patients cooperate with the therapist´s instructions for inspiratory exercises, strolling with aid, among others.

Follow-Up

Once these patients have left the hospital, they should be at least followed for one month, with another CT or chest X-ray, very likely with evidence of scarred tissue within the chest, but this is of no concern for the surgeon when the patient is asymptomatic. Rarely seen, are late complications of this disease, such would be the case of osteomyelitis of the ribs.

Complications

Unfortunately most patients with DNM eventually will develop complications related to the disease itself or the ICU, this is seen in 68-80% of the cases, the most commonly seen is pneumonia which is significantly more related to inferior DNM, in table 2 a summary of complications by author is demonstrated. [1,13,15]

Table 2. Complications according to different authors

Author (% of overall complications)	Complications
Ridder et al.,[1] (80%)	Pleural or pericardial effusion, pneumonia, septic shock, empyema, renal failure, arterial or vein thrombosis, multiple organ failure, arrhythmias, pericarditis, nerve paresis, cervical and thoracic fasciitis, acute respiratory distress syndrome, pneumothorax, swallowing disorders, fistulas, osteomyelitis, tracheomalacia and Lemier syndrome.
Deu-Martin et al.,[13] (58%)	Septic shock, heart failure, renal and/or hepatic failure, high digestive hemorrhage, cholecystitis, intestinal perforation, stroke and seizures.
Dajer-Fadel et al.,[15] (68%)	Pneumonia, septic shock, fistulas, empyema, multiple organ failure, cardiac arrest, acute renal insufficiency, pleural and/or pericardial effusion, air fistula, peneumothorax, wound dehiscence.

Since pneumonia is the most frequent, the authors hypothesized that tracheotomy played a role in the pathophysiology, out of 100 patients 74 were tracheotomized, this group had pneumonia 23% of the time, compared to 7.7% of the 26 cases that did not underwent this procedure, this difference has a borderline significant p value of 0.072, maybe because of the sample size, but definitely this issue has to be addressed during these patients´ management, and a review of the indications for tracheotomy clarified. [19] Every measure has to be taken to prevent or accurately treat these complications since they could clearly be a prelude to death.

Table 3. Main characteristics among the largest series of patients

Author	Year	No. of Patients	Mortality (%)
Ishinaga et al., [41]	2013	8	12
Bayarri Lara et al., [24]	2013	29	17.4
D´Cunha et al., [25]	2013	8	0
Cruz Toro et al., [26]	2013	6	0
Dajer-Fadel et al., [15]	2013	100	29
Ridder et al., [1]	2010	45	11.1
Deu-Martin et al., [13].	2010	43	21
Uwa et al., [27]	2009	5	0
Lin et al., [28]	2009	9	22
Chen et al., [29]	2008	18	16.7
Cho et al. [30]	2008	8	37.5
Roccia et al., [31]	2007	23	30.4
Misthos et al., [32]	2007	27	33.3
Sandner et al., [33]	2006	6	33.3
Iwata et al., [34]	2005	10	20
Papalia et al., [35]	2001	13	23
Freeman et al., [36]	2000	10	0
Sancho et al., [37]	1999	7	14
Marty-Ané et al., [38]	1999	12	16.5
Corsten et al., [39]	1997	8	12.5
Total		387	17.7

Prognosis

Interestingly, in recent years there have been a number of reports and patient series with less mortality rates than the past; as Ridder *et al.*[1] demonstrated in their meta-analysis comparing different periods: from 1960-1989 with 43 patients (34.9%), from 1990-1998 with 48 patients (22.9%), from 1999-2008 with 278 patients (15.5%) and their own results with 11.1% mortality, table 3 compares the mortality results in the last 16 years. Optimistically, when analyzing the low mortality rates with new surgical trends such as thoracoscopic surgery, a reduction in mortality is seen; a clear tendency towards this mode of treatment is envisioned around the world, some authors even report 0% mortality, however it is the authors´ opinion that a larger number of patients is needed to achieve reasonable conclusions. [39]

Table 4 summarizes the results from a thoracoscopic approach; it is fair to say that the latter technique is a feasible option, with comparable mortality and complication rates, however in patients with EP it may be difficult to repair by this technique.

Table 4. Analysis of recent literature regarding thoracoscopic approach. LOS = Lenght of stay, VATS = Video assited thoracoscopis surgery, DNM =Descending necrotizing mediastinitis, EP = Esophageal perforation

Author, date, journal and country	Main outcomes	Key results	Comments
Wakahara et al., [40] (2011), Asian Cardiovasc Thoac Surg, Japan	Mortality and hospital LOS with a minithoracotomy and thoracoscopic assistance	11 cases, LOS 30 – 117 days, mortality 0%	Mediastinum was opened longitudinally in at least 3 areas: anterior mediastinum, paratracheal space and posterior space of the trachea to the subcarinal space.
Ishinaga et al.,[41] (2013), Eur Arch Otorhinolaryngol, Japan	Compared VATS *vs.*mediastiniscopy, Mortality	8 cases treated, 6 by VATS, 2 by mediastinoscopy, mortality of 12%	9 out of 54 patients with deep cervical infection developed DNM, 1 patient was not treated by surgery
Cho et al., [30] (2008), Eur J Cardiothoracic Surg, Korea	VATS drainage, outcomes: symptom duration, progress, rate of conversion, mortality.	17 patients included, 9 for EP, 8 for cervical abscesses. Mean symptom duration was 12.4 days, hospital LOS 43.6, mortality 17.6%	Similar mortality rates than the open technique, however, 2 required conversion from complications of the original EP.

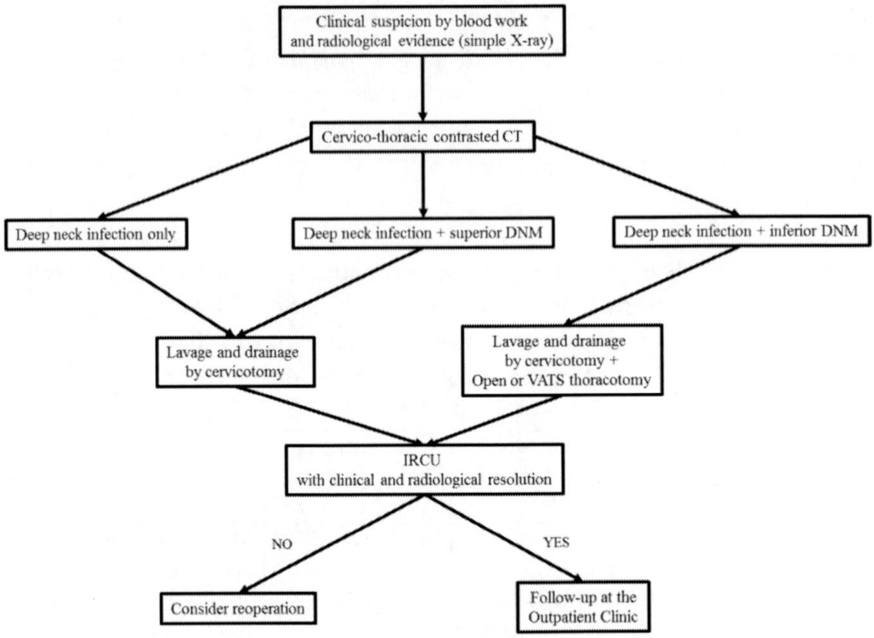

Figure 9. Proposed management algorithm for DNM by the authors. CT = computed tomography, DNM = descending necrotizing mediastinitis, IRCU = intensive respiratory care unit, VATS = video assisted thoracic surgery.

Conclusion

In recent years the number of reports have been growing considerably for this rare disease, as physicians gather more knowledge on the matter, hopefully mortality and morbidity will be reduced, the authors cannot emphasize enough the importance of early diagnosis, to achieve this, it is primordial to have a keen eye and quick suspicion that an odontogenic infection, a tonsillitis or even a skin infection could progress to a full blown mediastinitis, once diagnosis is evident, implementing a surgical plan is most important, never forgetting that in a whole, treatment for a patient with DNM is a multidisciplinary task; and as new technologies evolve, we could be hoping for better results and less complications. In Figure 9 a proposal for the management of DNM is shown summarizing what has been discussed in the chapter.

References

[1] Ridder GJ, Maier W, Kinzer S, Teszler CB, Boedeker CC, Pfeiffer J. Descending necrotizing mediastinitis: contemporary trends in etiology, diagnosis, management, and outcome. *Ann. Surg.* 2010;251(3):528-534.

[2] Dajer-Fadel WL, Ibarra-Pérez C, Sánchez-Velazquez LD, Borrego-Borrego R, Navarro-Reynoso FP, Argüero-Sánchez R. Descending necrotizing mediastinitis below the tracheal carina. *Asian Cardiovasc Thorac Ann* 2014;22(2):176-182.

[3] Sethi DS, Stanley RE. Deep neck abscesses—changing trends. *J Laryngol Otol* 1994;108(2):138-143.

[4] Suehara AB, Gonçalves AJ, Alcadipani FA, Kavabata NK, Menezes MB. Deep neck infection: analysis of 80 cases. *Braz J Otorhinolaryngol* 2008;74(2):253-259.

[5] Okten I, Cangir AK, Ozdemir N, Kavukçu S, Akay H, Yavuzer S. Management of esophageal perforation. *Surg Today* 2001;31(1):36-39.

[6] Bladergroen MR, Lowe JE, Postlethwait RW. Diagnosis and recommended management of esophageal perforation and rupture. *Ann Thorac Surg* 1986;42(3):235-239.

[7] Johnson SB. Esophageal trauma. *Semin Thorac Cardiovasc Surg* 2008;20:46-51.

[8] Dajer-Fadel WL, Borrego-Borrego R, Flores-Calderon O, Ibarra-Perez C. Descending necrotizing mediastinitis and thoracic cellulitis due to varicella. *Asian Cardiovasc Thorac Ann* 2012;20(1):83-85.

[9] Dajer-Fadel WL, Borrego-Borrego R, Flores-Calderón O, Argüero-Sánchez R, Navarro-Reynoso FP, Ibarra-Pérez C. Descending necrotizing mediastinitis associated with spinal cord abscess. *Asian Cardiovasc Thorac Ann* 2013;21(1):90-92.

[10] Dajer-Fadel WL, Ibarra-Pérez C, Borrego-Borrego R, Navarro-Reynoso FP, Argüero-Sánchez R. Descending necrotizing mediastinitis and sternoclavicular joint osteomyelitis. *Asian Cardiovasc Thorac Ann* 2013;21(5):618-620.

[11] Dajer-Fadel WL, Ibarra-Perez C, Borrego-Borrego R, Flores-Calderon O. Thoracic necrotizing fasciitis due to snake ointment that progressed to a mediastinitis. *Interact Cardiovasc Thorac Surg* 2012;14(1):94-95.

[12] Brook I, Frazier EH. Microbiology of mediastinitis. *Arch Intern Med* 1996;156:333-336.

[13] Deu-Martin M, Saez-Barba M, López-Sanz I, Alcaraz-Peñarrocha R, Romero-Vielva L, Solé-Montserrat J. Factores de riesgo de mortalidad

en la mediastinitis necrosante descendente. *Arch Bronconeumol* 2010;46:182-187.

[14] Shields TW: Primary tumors and cysts of the mediastinum. In: Shields TW, ed. General Thoracic Surgery, Philadelphia: Lea & Febiger, 1972:908.

[15] Dajer-Fadel W, Ibarra-Pérez C, Solís-Suarez J, Sánchez-Velázquez L, Tortolero-Sánchez C, Borrego-Borrego R, Navarro-Reynoso F, Argüero-Sánchez R. Superior and Inferior Descending Necrotizing Mediastinitis, 100 cases. *Chest* 2013;144:117A-117A.

[16] Estrera AS, Lanay MJ, Grisham JM, Sinn DP, Platt MR. Descending necrotizing mediastinitis. *Surg Gynecol Obstet* 1983;157:545-552.

[17] Capps EF, Kinsella JJ, Gupta M, Bhatki AM, Opatowsky MJ. Emergency imaging assessment of acute, non-traumatic conditions of the head and neck. *Radiographics* 2010;30:1335-1352.

[18] Endo S, Murayama F, Hasegawa T, Yamamoto S, Yamaguchi T, Sohara Y, Fuse K, Miyata M, Nishino H. Guideline of surgical management based on diffusion of descending necrotizing mediastinitis. *Jpn J Thorac Cardiovasc Surg* 1999;47(1):14-19.

[19] Falcoz PE. The Thoracic Surgery Scoring System (Thoracoscore): risk model for in-hospital death in 15,183 patients requiring thoracic surgery. *J Thoracic Cardiovasc Surg* 2007;133:325-332.

[20] Chamogeorgakis TP. Thoracoscore predicts midterm mortality in patients undergoing thoracic surgery. *J Thorac Cardiovasc Surg* 2007;134:883-887.

[21] Chamogeorgakis T. External validation of the modified thoracoscore in a new thoracic surgery program: prediction of in-hospital mortality. *Interact Cardiovasc Thorac Surg* 2009;9:463-466.

[22] Metnitz PG, Moreno RP, Almeida E, Jordan B, Bauer P, Campos RA, Iapichino G, Edbrooke D, Capuzzo M, Le Gall JR; SAPS 3 Investigators. SAPS 3-From evaluation of the patient to evaluation of the intensive care unit. Part 1: Objectives, methods and cohort description. *Intensive Care Med* 2005;31:1336-1344.

[23] Moreno RP, Metnitz PG, Almeida E, Jordan B, Bauer P, Campos RA, Iapichino G, Edbrooke D, Capuzzo M, Le Gall JR; SAPS 3 Investigators. SAPS 3-From evaluation of the patient to evaluation of the intensive care unit. Part 2: Development of a prognostic model for hospital mortality at ICU admission. *Intensive Care Med* 2005;31:1345-1355.

[24] Bayarri Lara CI, Sevilla López S, Sánchez-Palencia Ramos A, Alkourdi Martínez A, Hernández Escobar F, Quero Valenzuela F, Ruiz Zafra FJ, Cueto Ladrón de Guevara A. Surgical management of descending necrotizing mediastinitis. *Cir Esp* 2013;91(9):579-583.
[25] D'Cunha J, James M, Antonoff MB, Green CA, Andrade RS, Maddaus MA, Beilman GJ. Descending necrotizing mediastinitis: a modified algorithmic approach to define a new standard of care. *Surg Infect (Larchmt)* 2013;14(6):525-531.
[26] Cruz Toro P, Callejo Castillo A, Tornero Saltó J, González Compta X, Farré A, Maños M. Cervical necrotizing fasciitis: Report of 6 cases and review of literature. *Eur Ann Otorhinolaryngol Head Neck Dis* 2014;14:S1879-7296.
[27] Uwa N, Terada T, Saeki N, Sagawa K, Ogino K, Sakagami M. Clinical features of 5 patients with descending necrotizing mediastinitis originating from deep neck infection. *Auris Nasus Larynx* 2010;37(4):530-534.
[28] Lin CX, Ding X, Ma YK, Zhang XF, Zhu XH. Infections of the head and neck leading to descending necrotizing mediastinitis: management of 9 cases. *Zhonghua Kou Qiang Yi Xue Za Zhi* 2009;44(10):619-620.
[29] Chen KC, Chen JS, Kuo SW, Huang PM, Hsu HH, Lee JM, Lee YC. Descending necrotizing mediastinitis: a 10-year surgical experience in a single institution. *J Thorac Cardiovasc Surg* 2008;136(1):191-198.
[30] Cho JS, Kim YD, IH, Lee SK, Jeong YJ. Treatment of mediastinitis using videoassisted thoracic surgery. *Eur J Cardiothorac Surg* 2008;34:520-524.
[31] Roccia F, Pecorari GC, Oliaro A, Passet E, Rossi P, Nadalin J, Garzino-Demo P, Berrone S. Ten years of descending necrotizing mediastinitis: Management of 23 cases. *J Oral Maxillofac Surg* 2007;65:1716-1724.
[32] Misthos P, Katsagarakis S, Kakaris S, Theodorou D, Skottis I. Descending necrotizing mediastinitis: Analysis of survival and surgical treatment modalities. *J Oral Maxillofac Surg* 2007;65:635-639.
[33] Sandner A, Börgermann J, Kosling S, Bloching MB. Descending necrotizing mediastinitis due to deep neck infections. Incidence and management. *HNO* 2006;54:861-867.
[34] Iwata T, Sekine Y, Shibuya K, Yasufuku K, Iyoda A, Iizasa T, Saito Y, Fujisawa T. Early open thoracotomy and mediastinopleural irrigation for severe descending necrotizing mediastinitis. *Eur J Cardiothorac Surg* 2005;28:384-388.

[35] Papalia E, Rena O, Oliaro A, Cavallo A, Giobbe R, Casadio C, Maggi G, Mancuso M. Descending necrotizing mediastinitis: surgical management. *Eur J Cardiothorac Surg* 2001;20:739-742.

[36] Freeman RK, Vallieres E, Verrier ED, Karmy-Jones R, Wood DE. Desending necrotizing mediastinitis: an analysis of the effects of serial surgical debridement on patient mortality. *J Thorac Cardiovasc Surg* 2000;119:260-267.

[37] Sancho LMM, Minamoto H, Fernandez A, Sennes LU, Jatene FB. Descending necrotizing mediastinitis: a retrospective surgical experience. *Eur J Cardiothorac Surg* 1999;16:200-205.

[38] Marty-Ané C-H, Berthet J-P, Alric P, Pegis JD, Rouvière P, Mary H. Management of descending necrotizing mediastinitis: An aggressive treatment for an aggressive disease. *Ann Thorac Surg* 1999;68:212-217.

[39] Corsten MJ, Shamji FM, Odell PF, Frederico JA, Laframboise GG, Reid KR, Vallieres E, Matzinger F. Optimal treatment of descending necrotizing mediastinitis. *Thorax* 1997;52:702-708.

[40] Wakahara T, Tanaka Y, Maniwa Y, Nishio W, Yoshimura M. Successful management of descending necrotizing mediastinitis. *Asian Cardiovasc Thorac Ann* 2011;19(3-4):228-231.

[41] Ishinaga H, Otsu K, Sakaida H, Miyamura T, Nakamura S, Kitano M, Tempaku H, Takao M, Kobayashi, Takeuchi K. Descending necrotizing mediastinitis from deep neck infection. *Eur Arch Otorhinolaryngol.* 2013;270(4):1463-1466.

In: Mediastinal Infections
Editor: Walid Leonardo Dajer-Fadel
ISBN: 978-1-63463-369-7

Chapter 4

Correlative Anatomy in Descending Necrotizing Mediastinitis

***W. L. Dajer-Fadel*[1*], *A. Munguía-Félix*[2] *and G. Campos-Bolaños*[2]**

[1] Cardiothoracic Surgery Department, General Hospital of Mexico "Dr. Eduardo Liceaga", Mexico City, Mexico

[2] Radiology Department, General Hospital of Mexico "Dr. Eduardo Liceaga", Mexico City, Mexico

Abstract

Radiological imaging is essential for the diagnosis of descending necrotizing mediastinitis (DNM), a contrast-enhanced CT of the cervical and thoracic regions is the study considered the standard of care, it helps to evaluate and look for the presence of adipose tissue heterogeneity, gas bubbles, air-fluid levels, abscessed fluid collections, pneumo-mediastinum, pneumopericardium, subcutaneous emphysema, and pericardial or pleural effusion in the context of a patient with a cervical or upper thoracic infection; it is important to identify the normal anatomy, mediastinal spaces and zones to properly separate superior -above tracheal carina- and inferior – above and below tracheal carina- signs of

* Correspondence to: Walid Leonardo Dajer-Fadel, E-mail address: drdajer@gmail.com.

DNM. Once these steps are done properly, a sound decision can be made to complete their treatment protocol. The chapter will present a pictorial essay for a proper diagnostic workup in DNM, based on representative CT images of patients treated with this disease.

Introduction

Mediastinal infections are classified as acute or chronic, the first can be of three different types, such as descending, post-operative and ascending, while the latter are classified as fibrosing or granulomatous mediastinitis due to chronic or idiopathic diseases. Sometimes diagnosis of the acute descending type results difficult for surgeons and clinicians alike, because in some occasions simple chest x-rays are not clear, leading to a delay in patient management, that is why now days the tool of choice as standard of care is a contrast-enhanced CT (CECT) where the spaces formed between the fascia can be seen when affected by an infectious process, in occasions, it is very evident, and in others even expert radiologists have a hard time concluding a diagnosis of DNM. It is the authors´ belief that a CECT should always be performed when treating patients with deep neck or upper thoracic infections that have the potential to advance into deeper planes and produce DNM, because an infection rarely seems to be confined to the cervical level when it has already advanced to mediastinal zones, and if no attention is put into this, catastrophic results may arise. In this chapter a review is offered regarding diagnostic imaging in patients with DNM for any of its causes, also postoperative relevant information regarding surgical decisions when re-operating a patient.

Spaces That Lead to the Mediastinum

As seen in previous chapters, the fascia from where an infectious process can spread from the neck or superficial layers of the upper chest into the mediastinal zones have been explained, in figure 1 a correlative MRI image shows the most important spaces that play a role in the spread of disease.

It is important to understand that in occasions they are considered as "virtual spaces" because of their potential to become real areas that harvest purulent exudate that could accumulate in great quantities unless they are drained.

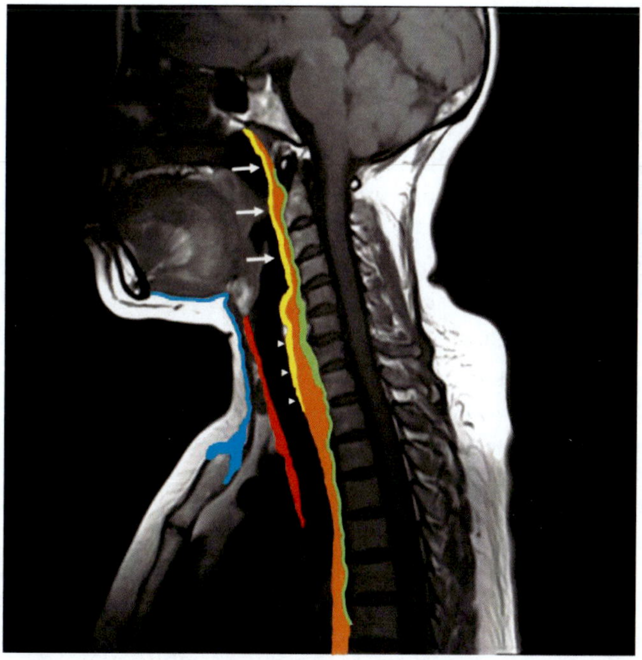

Figure 1. Sagittal magnetic resonance of the cervico-thoracic regions demonstrating the potential spaces for a descending necrotizing mediastinitis when propagating into the mediastinum, these are the suprasternal (*blue*), pre-tracheal (*red*) and retropharyngeal (*yellow with arrows*) spaces that continues as the retro-visceral or retroesophageal (*yellow with arrowheads*) space; also the dangerous space (*orange*) and the prevertebral space (*green*) are depicted.

In a gross manner, infections that involve the suprasternal and pre-tracheal spaces, eventually dissect the prevascular zone; carotid space abscesses affect the visceral and retrovisceral zones; and finally, the retro-esophageal, danger, and prevetebral spaces involve the retrovisceral zone in the majority of cases.

Endo *et al.* as mentioned in chapter 1 divided DNM in three types based on their radiological appearance according to spread of infection (Figure 2), however it is the authors´ opinion that it is inaccurate for various reasons: a) the classification was done based on only 4 patients, b) making a distinction between types IIA and IIB has no clinical, prognostic or management implications, and c) there is no way to classify the disease when the pericardium and its contents are affected. As expected, many authors do make a distinction between the superior and inferior types, having as point of reference the tracheal carina (Figure 3), some have not found a mortality difference, however, it helped to make accurate surgical decisions as to perform only a cervicotomy or a cervicotomy plus a thoracotomy; the authors did find a significant difference with lower mortality for patients with superior DNM against inferior DNM (10.3 *vs* 36,6% p = 0.006). [1, 2]

It has been suggested that for type I DNM, patients should receive only cervical drainage, for Type IIA a cervical plus subxiphoid approach and for type IIB, cervicotomy plus thoracotomy. [1] However others have studied the best approach to mediastinal infections below the tracheal carina and concluded that for the inferior type a thoracotomy plus cervicotomy is the only and best surgery a patient could be offered. [2, 3] Endo´s Classification proved inaccurate in a study made by Kwang Kang et al., where out of 56 patients with deep cervical infections (DNI), 12 had DNM and all were classified as type IIB receiving a thoracotomy as treatment of choice in, accordance to other authors that also suggest this as the best approach. [4]

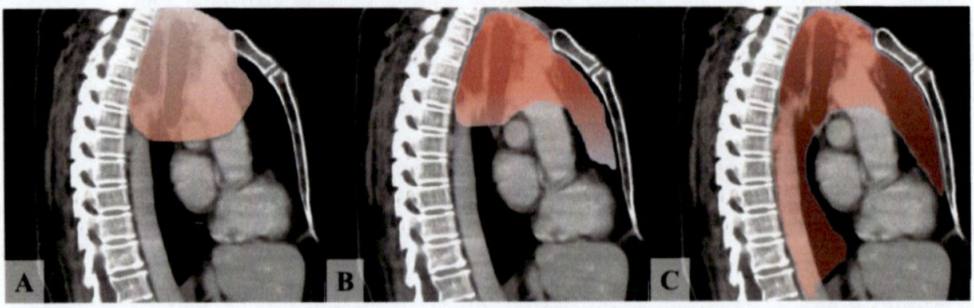

Figure 2. Endo´s classification viewed with a sagittal reconstruction during contrast-enhanced computed tomography: (A) Type I, (B) Type IIA and (C) Type IIB.

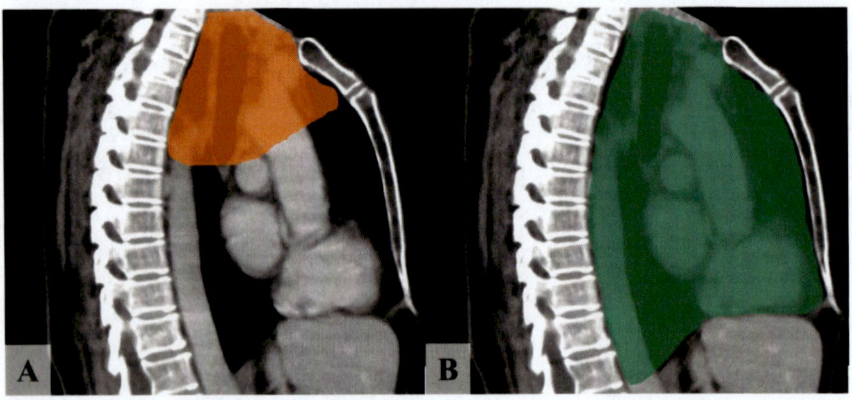

Figure 3. Simple classification proposed by the authors as: (A) Superior descending necrotizing mediastinitis and (B) Inferior descending necrotizing mediastinitis.

Simple Cervical and Chest X-Ray

It is well known that a CECT is the standard of care in patients with DNM, however two situations are worth mentioning; since not all first contact physicians have a CT scanner available, it is important to know how to identify simple x-ray abnormalities at the cervical and thoracic levels to know when to refer a patient to an institution that has a Thoracic Surgery Department. Also, some physicians believe that it is excessive to order a chest CT scan to every patient with a DNI, so performing a simple chest x-ray will have to suffice or evaluate the need for a CT scan through this study. Hernández-Aranda et al. analyzed the correlation between simple X-rays and CT scans in patients with DNI and DNM, they had 18 patients (out of 30) with a DNI and suspicion of DNM that where confirmed with the disease when checked with a CT scan; the simple X-ray signs compatible with DNM in patients with DNI are: a) mediastinal widening, b) bilateral or left para-cardiac air lines, c) mediastinal widening plus paracardiac air lines, and d) heterogeneity of the supra-aortic tissues plus air in the shape of bands in the para-cardiac mediastinum; out of the 12 patients that did not have DNM by CT, four also presented mediastinal widening in simple chest X-rays but no correlation could be seen on CT. According to the authors all patients that had DNM also had some sign on simple chest x-rays, therefore this study demonstrated a high specificity (100%) when no signs are found; however mediastinal widening resulted with a 77% sensitivity and a 66% specificity, however, when other signs are found with widened mediastinum, such as pneumomediastinum, the diagnosis of DNM is very suggestive, concluding that in the absence of signs in simple chest X-rays, DNM could be discarded, unfortunately this is the only study that has analyzed this correlation. [5]

In some cases, DNM is caused by an esophageal perforation where fluid levels, pneumothorax and pneumomediastinum may be seen, confirmed by esophagograms, remembering that these have 10-25% rates of false negative results, it is important to avoid using barium because of the possibility of barium-induced mediastinal inflammation, water-soluble contrast is preferred. Other important signs are pericardial or pleural effusion. [6]

Simple X-rays have a very limited use, however they serve a great role in the initial study protocol performed to patients with suspected DNM to decide whether or not to proceed with tomography. The most important limitation is the inability to produce high quality images, so a surgical procedure could be planned, reason for which CT gained more acceptance.

Computed Tomography

This has proven once and again to be a great diagnostic tool; it allows physicians to evaluate thoroughly the cervical and thoracic anatomy helping clarify the extension of DNM, more importantly, above or below the tracheal carina, also, it is much more sensitive than any other method. Many authors have published several findings associated to DNM such as fluid collections, gas, pericardial and pleural effusions, soft tissue edema and heterogeniety of the mediastinal adipose tissue. [7] Deu-Martín *et al.* reported 43 patients treated for DNM, from which 51.7% had mediastinal fat infiltration, 29.7% defined abscesses (enhanced by contrast material in their borders) and 18.9% with air bubbles. Regarding the extension of disease, superior DNM was seen in 85.5% and inferior DNM in 14.5%. [8] This contrasts with what the authors have found which is 29% for the first and 71% for the latter. [2]

Based on what has been reviewed, in superior DNM tomographic signs are going to be equivalent to the area affected, due to the virtual spaces found in the area, air bubbles could appear because of proliferation of gas-producing anaerobe bacteria; regarding adipose and connective tissue surrounding the great vessels, trachea and esophagus, infiltration of the infectious process could exist with subsequent edema of soft tissues, translating it as heterogeneity of the mediastinal fat; as infection advances, it may produce a purulent discharge between the spaces, seen as air-fluid levels, heterogenic collections with contrast-enhanced walls, suggesting well formed abscesses, making these the most common findings in this type of DNM (Figures 4–11).

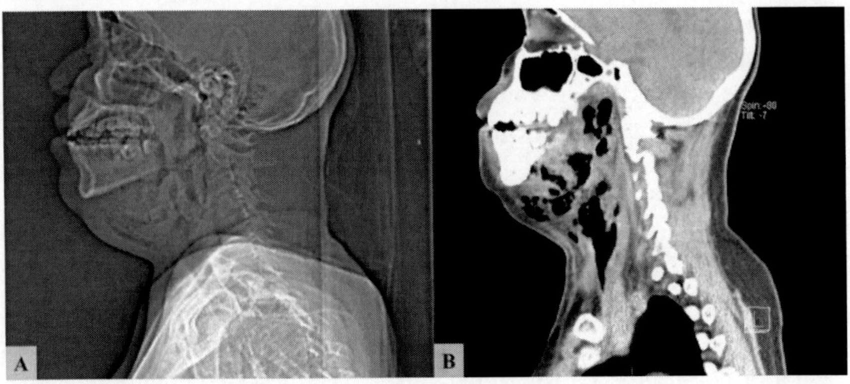

Figure 4. (A) Lateral view of a cervical scanogram of patient with a deep neck gas-producing abscess showed as low density regions within the collection and a swelling neck, in the sagittal tomographic view (B) gas bubbles are more evident.

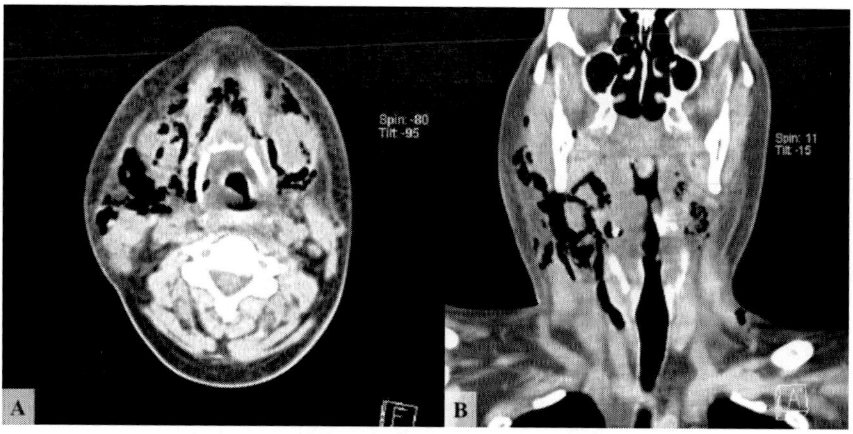

Figure 5. (A) Axial and (B) coronal cervical computed tomography of patient with gas dissecting to both anterior and left posterior cervical triangles from a right deep neck abscess limited to the superior mediastinum and neck, gas and heterogeneity of adipose tissue can be seen.

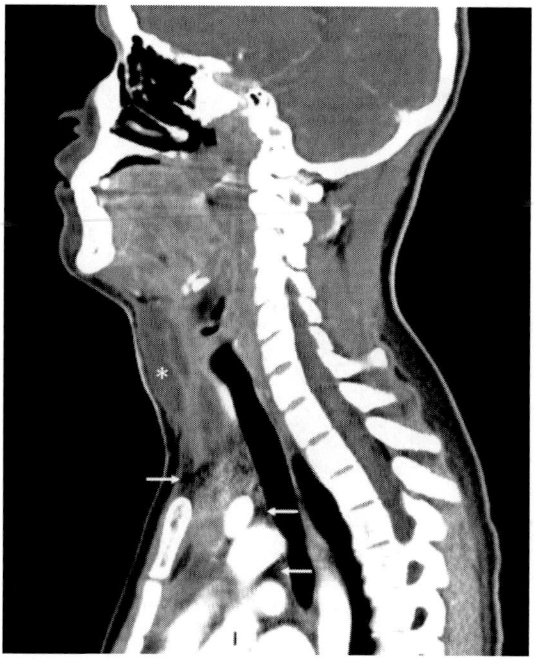

Figure 6. Sagittal contrast-enhanced cervical tomography of a patient with a superficial anterior abscess in the right anterior triangle (*asterisk*) where hypodense collections can be seen, immediately inferior to the lesion, heterogeneity of adipose tissue and gas in the suprasternal space are seen, also in the pre-tracheal spacc (*arrows*).

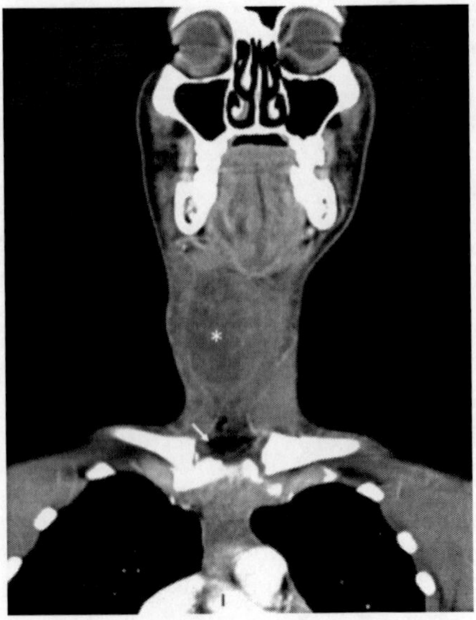

Figure 7. Same patient as figure 6 where in the coronal view, a more evident anterior abscess (*asterisk*) is seen with the underlying gas bubbles (*arrow*).

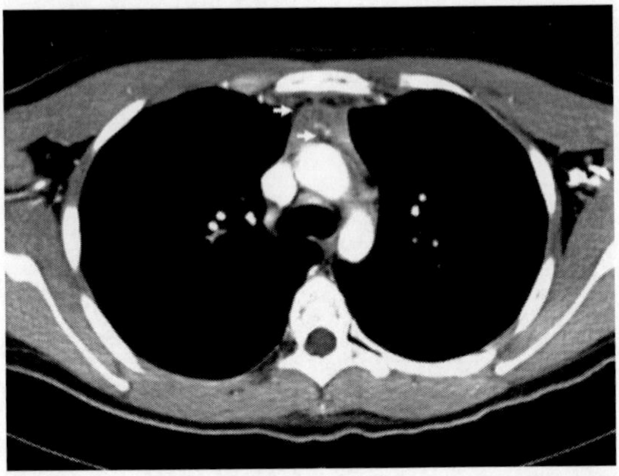

Figure 8. Male patient with superior descending necrotizing mediastinitis with gas bubbles (*arrows*) in the pre-vascular zone above the tracheal carina.

However, the disease is always prone to advance and dissect more to caudal planes, spaces and tissues, progressing to an inferior DNM; corresponding findings due to exudate and fluid extension, pleural or pericardial effusions could be seen; and when anaerobes are involved, pneumomediastinum or pneumopericardium are present; rarely subcutaneous emphysema is present (Figures 12-14). It is important to remark, when DNM is due to an esophageal perforation, gas may not be secondary to anaerobes, but from migration of the mentioned viscera where subcutaneous emphysema is much more evident, and rarely, pneumothorax could also be seen (Figures 15,16).

Once diagnosis is suspected, correlating any of the previously mentioned signs, backed up by clinical data and history of disease, a consensus is made between the surgeons and clinicians to decide the most reasonable treatment plan; when DNM is evident, invariably surgery should be undertaken.

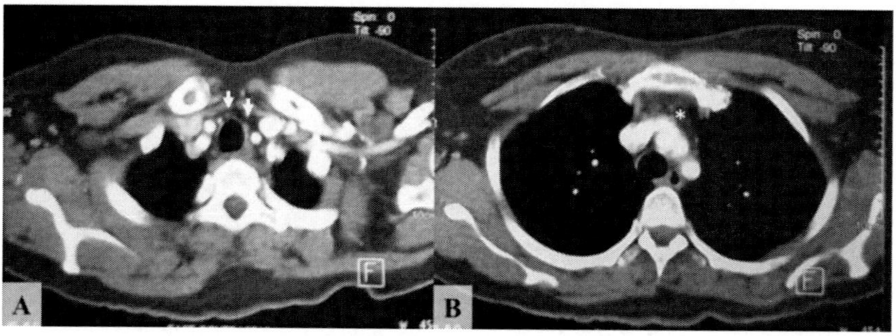

Figure 9. Axial contrast-enhanced tomographic views of at the suprasternal level (A) and in the mediastinum above the tracheal carina (B) where gas dissection (*arrows*) is seen followed with heterogeneity (*asterisk*) of the pre-vascular zone´s adipose tissue in a patient with superior descending necrotizing mediastinitis.

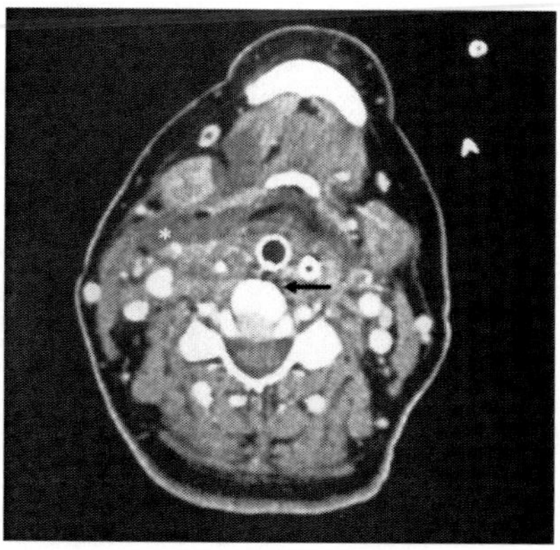

Figure 10. Axial cervical contrast-enhanced tomography in a patient with superior descending necrotizing mediastinitis with a right abscess (*asterisk*) demonstrating a hypodense image suggestive of exudate surrounded by edematous tissues. Also peri-esophageal gas can be seen (*black arrow*).

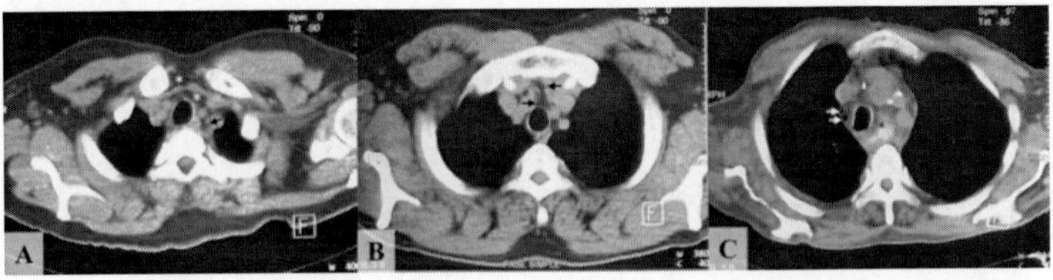

Figure 11. Contrast-enhanced axial tomographic view of patient with superior descending necrotizing mediastinitis, from A to C gas dissection is seen from the supra-sternal notch (*asterisks*), the retrosternal area (*black arrows*) and right lower tracheal region (*white arrows*). Notice a true image of heterogeneity within the great vessels (*triangle*).

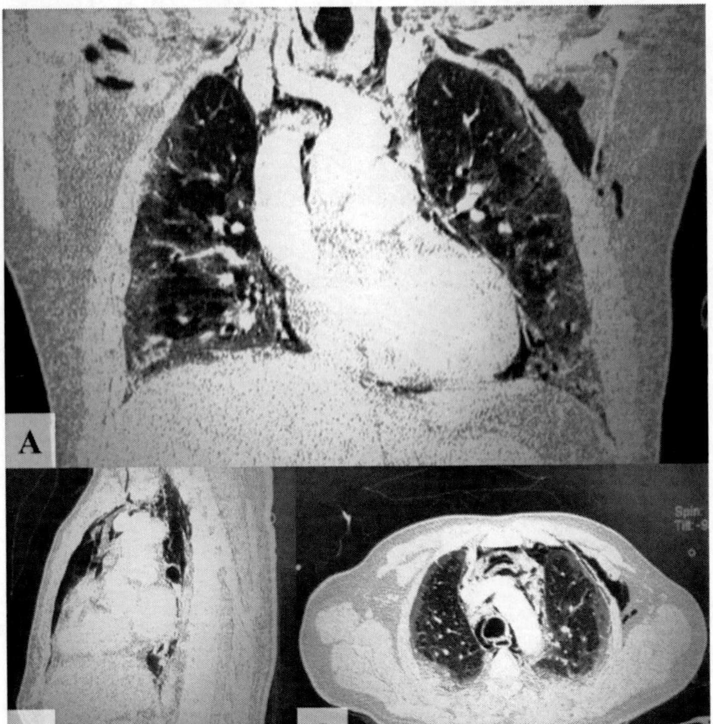

Figure 12. Computed tomography in the parenchymal window of patient with an overwhelming inferior descending necrotizing mediastinitis with extensive tissue dissection within the perivascular, para-cardiac, retro-esophageal and subcutaneous tissues in the coronal (A), sagittal (B) and axial (C) views.

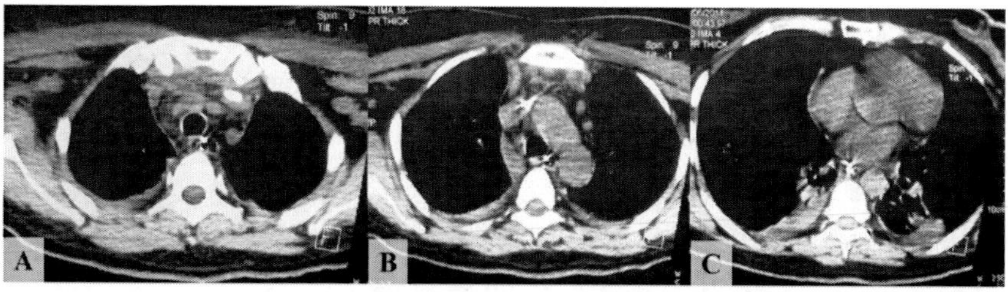

Figure 13. Mediastinal window CT of patient with an inferior type mediastinitis demonstrating adipose tissue heterogeneity, gas bubbles in the same area and the retro-visceral space followed by bilateral pleural effusions in various levels from the mediastinum above the tracheal carina (A,B), and below it (C).

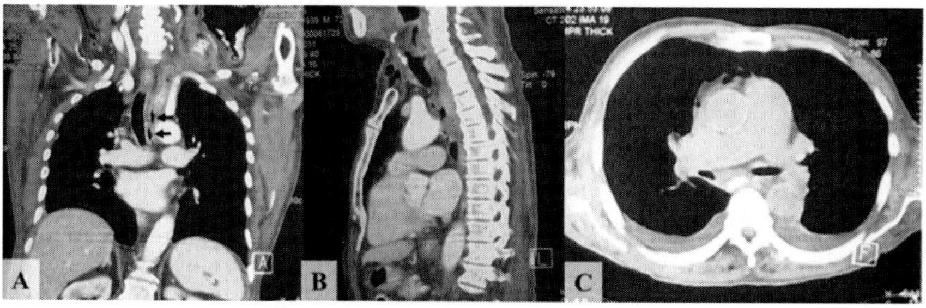

Figure 14. Contrast-enhanced computed tomography of patient with inferior descending necrotizing mediastinitis in the (A) coronal view demonstrating para-tracheal gas (*arrows*), also edema, exudate and gas could be seen in the retro-esophageal space in the sagittal view (B), finally bilateral pleural effusion was evident (C) in the inferior axial view.

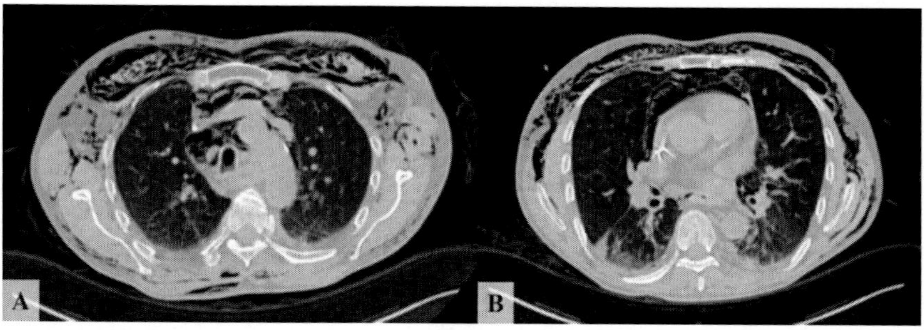

Figure 15. Axial tomographic view of the mediastinum above (A) and below (B) the tracheal carina of a patient that sustained an esophageal perforation followed by overwhelming subcutaneous emphysema, wide pneumomediastinum with a bilateral pleural effusion and pneumopericardium.

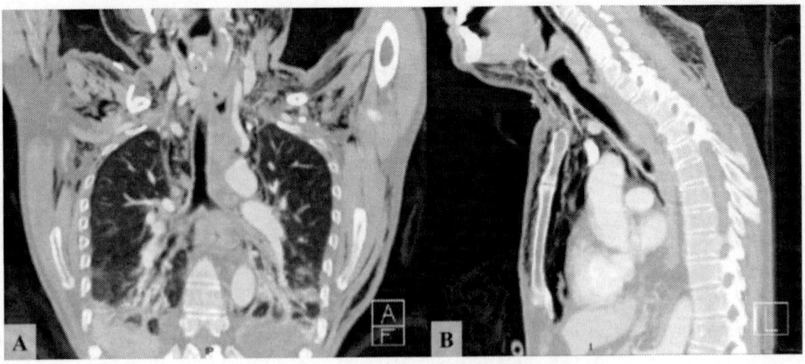

Figure 16. Same patient as figure 15 where in the coronal (A) and sagittal (B) views a clear dissection is seen among the mentioned tissues and spaces.

Post-Operative Imaging

Follow-up is very important because in many occasions a re-evaluation is needed to determine if the patient would benefit from a second or more interventions because of an unsatisfactory progression of disease, seen by leukocytosis persistence and other indicators of sepsis. In the author's review, 13.3% of the patients needed a second thoracotomy 12.7 ± 6.5 (range 6-19) days after the first surgery, four for persistent empyema, three for CT-evident residual mediastinal abscesses, and one for necrotizing pneumonia, 3 (37.5%) of this sub-group died. [9]

Several authors believe a CT scan should be performed routinely every 48 hours until disease improves, [10,11] however it is also justified to perform it 72 hours post-operatively or even doing only serial simple chest X-rays, and a CT only in cases when there is inadequate progression of disease. Unfortunately no randomized controlled trials have been performed on the matter, most likely due to the scarce number of available patients.

In occasions just by looking at the images one could be fooled of the disease´s severity, that is why it is so important to pay attention to the patient´s current clinical situation, where, if there is adequate progression of the infectious process with decreased post-operative leukocytes, fever absence, an awake patient and serous fluid in the drainages, but CT scan still has pleural effusion or heterogeneity of adipose tissue, a strong consideration should be made to not operate. On the other hand, if same scenario appears but with turbid drainage, fever or leukocytosis, surgery should be performed (Figures 17, 18).

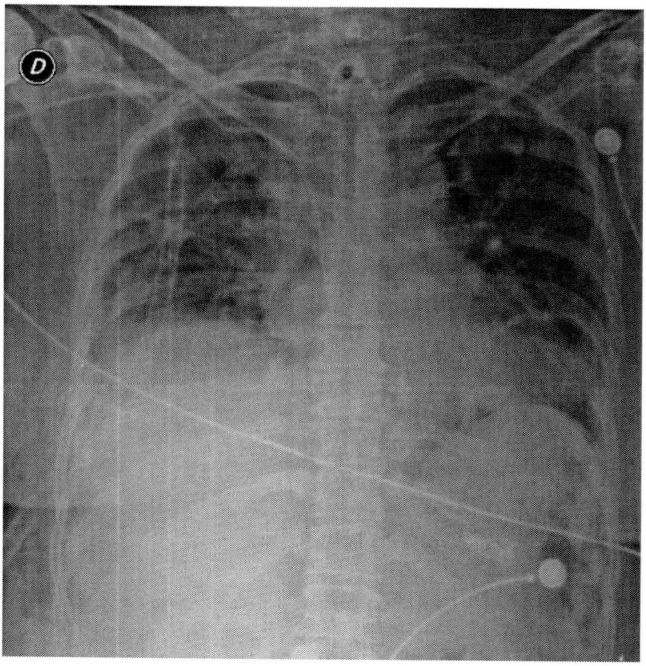

Figure 17. Simple chest x-ray taken just after a transthoracic drainage and lavage of the mediastinum was performed, demonstrating two right and one left chest tubes for post-operative control.

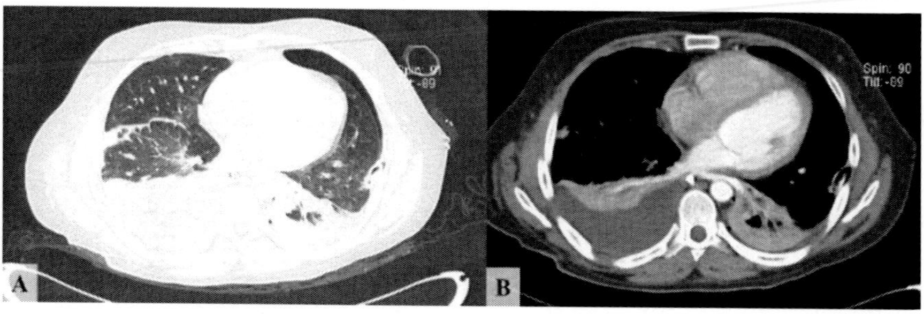

Figure 18. Contrast-enhanced tomography in the parenchymal (A) and mediastinal (B) windows of a patient 10 days after drainage and lavage for DNM, where a moderate right pleural effusion could be seen due to early right chest tube removal, also a left pneumothorax is evident with a malfunctioning drainage. This patient only required a new right chest tube and re-permeabilization of the left tube with continued antibiotic therapy.

Conclusion

In many occasions it is hard to make a decision to whether extend or not the time of mediastinal drainage and lavage based on radiographic findings, most of the time the signs of extension into the mediastinum below the level of the tracheal carina are not quite clear, it is the authors´ opinion that since this is a disease of fatal consequences when not operated upon, the surgeon should have a very sensible threshold for deciding to whether operate the thoracic cavity and mediastinal zones or not, however, it is preferable to find out to be mistaken during surgery than not performing the procedure when the mediastinum was truly affected, and see before his eyes patients that are too late or their risk factors for mortality have increased, after trying a conservative approach.

It is very important to pay attention to clinical data as well as radiological imaging. A contrast-enhanced cervico-thoracic CT in mediastinal window mode is still the standard of care when diagnosing this disease, and if by any reason contrast materials can´t be infused, it is still justified to perform a simple CT.

References

[1] Endo S, Murayama F, Hasegawa T, Yamamoto S, Yamaguchi T, Sohara Y, Fuse K, Miyata M, Nishino H. Guideline of surgical management based on diffusion of descending necrotizing mediastinitis. *Jpn J Thorac Cardiovasc Surg* 1999;47(1):14-19.

[2] Dajer-Fadel WL, Ibarra-Pérez C, Solís-Suárez JA, Sánchez-Velázquez LD, Tortolero-Sánchez C, Borrego-Borrego R, Navarro-Reynoso FP, Argüero-Sánchez, R. Superior and inferior descending necrotizing mediastinitis, 100 cases. *Chest* 2013;144,117A-117A.

[3] Misthos P, Katsaragakis S, Kakaris S, Theodorou D, Skottis I. Descending necrotizing anterior mediastinitis: analysis of survival and surgical treatment modalities. *J. Oral Maxillofac Surg* 2007;65(4):635-639.

[4] Kwang SK, Lee S, Oh HK, Kang MW, Yu JH, Koo BS, Lim SP. Clinical features of deep neck infections and predisposing factors for mediastinal extension. *Korean J Thorac Cardiovasc Surg* 2012;45(3):171-176.

[5] Hernández Aranda JA, Guerrero Avedaño G. Correlación de hallazgos por radiología convencional y tomografía computada en la extensión mediastinal secundaria a absceso profundo de cuello: utilidad de la radiografía de tórax. *An Radiol Mex* 2011;3:167-173.

[6] Goldstein LA, Thompson WR. Esophageal perforation: a 15-year experience. *Am J Surg* 1992;143:495-503.

[7] Boiselle PhM. Diffuse mediastinal abnormalities. In: McLoud ThC, editor. *Thoracic radiology, the requisites.* St Louis (MO): Mosby; 1998. P. 464-467.

[8] Deu-Martín M1, Saez-Barba M, López Sanz I, Alcaraz Peñarrocha R, Romero Vielva L, Solé Montserrat J. Mortality risk factors in descending necrotizing mediastinitis. *Arch Bronconeumol* 2010;46(4):182-187.

[9] Dajer-Fadel WL, Ibarra-Pérez C, Sánchez-Velazquez LD, Borrego-Borrego R, Navarro-Reynoso FP, Argüero-Sánchez R. Descending necrotizing mediastinitis below the tracheal carina. *Asian Cardiovasc Thorac Ann* 2014;22(2):176-182.

[10] De Freitas RP, Fahy CP, Brooker DS, Primrose WJ, McManus KG, McGuigan JA, Hughes SJ. Descending necrotising mediastinitis: a safe treatment algorithm. *Eur Arch Otorhinolaryngol* 2007;264(2):181-187.

[11] Freeman RK, Vallières E, Verrier ED, Karmy-Jones R, Wood DE. Descending necrotizing mediastinitis: An analysis of the effects of serial surgical debridement on patient mortality. *J Thorac Cardiovasc Surg* 2000;119(2):260-267.

In: Mediastinal Infections
Editor: Walid Leonardo Dajer-Fadel
ISBN: 978-1-63463-369-7

Chapter 5

Surgical Management for Descending Necrotizing Mediastinitis

W. L. Dajer-Fadel*
Cardiothoracic Surgery Department, General Hospital of Mexico "Dr. Eduardo Liceaga", Mexico City, Mexico

Abstract

Mediastinal drainage is the cornerstone for the treatment of descending necrotizing mediastinitis (DNM), many options have emerged throughout the years to adequately drain and lavage the spaces comprised by it. Definitely a right thoracotomy has been the most widely used technique allowing the surgeon to approach the retrovisceral, visceral and prevascular zones with ease, however other incisions such as transsternal, clamshell, subxiphoid or bilateral thoracotomies have been proposed without much success. Minimally invasive surgery has been gaining terrain in the past years, a procedure that most probably will substitute traditional approaches. Invariably of the thoracic incision, a cervicotomy should be performed in all cases. The chapter will review all the available surgical options for the management of these patients.

* Correspondence to: Walid Leonardo Dajer-Fadel, E-mail address: drdajer@gmail.com.

Introduction

Since the work of Pierce [1] in 1938 where a thorough description comparing patients that did not undergo surgical debridement for DNM against a group that did, reported a mortality reduction from 86% to 35% in the operated group; surgery has become the standard of care for patients with this disease. However, the best approach for the varying cases and etiologies has always been debated until this day without reaching a consensus to appropriately guide surgeons. [2-4] Some evidence has been published regarding suggested techniques, but there is still a need for prospective studies that would help determine this decision. Many ways for drainage and lavage of the mediastinum have been described, such as cervical, subxiphoid, thoracotomy and clamshell incisions, or a mixture of them. In 1997 Roberts et al. described the first thoracoscopic approach to drain and treat mediastinal infections in a 69 year-old patient. [5] As medicine becomes as minimally invasive as possible in recent years, this technique has gained acceptance but it´s still the standard of care for which a right thoracotomy has the domain. The chapter offers a review of all the techniques with a more thorough description of right thoracotomy and thoracoscopic methods.

Right Thoracotomy

This technique by far is the most utilized by thoracic surgeons around the globe, in many occasions, transthoracic approach has been suggested to be performed regardless of the extension of mediastinal disease. [6-8] It is the authors belief that this method is ideal for an adequate and thorough dissection of the three mediastinal zones and the contralateral thoracic cavity (through the same incision), it also allows to permeabilize the retroesophageal and retropharyngeal spaces, communicating the original cervical abscess downwards so that no fluid remains static, allowing antibiotics to counteract the impending infectious process with more ease. In the following lines, a description of the steps undertaken to perform this surgery is explained.

With the patient selectively intubated to the left a right lung collapse is achieved, allowing unobstructed visualization of the right mediastinal pleura. It is always recommendable to place a naso-gastric tube so that the esophagus could be clearly identified during the procedure because this structure is prone to lesions due to its friability and altered structural micro- and macroscopical anatomy. Positioning of the body is done in a left decubitus manner; a folded blanket on the down side or flexing the operating table just above the iliac crest will allow opening of the ribs to facilitate maneuverability of the thoracic cavity.

Once the patient is in position, antisepsis is performed; a right posterolateral thoracotomy is done with a traditional or muscle sparing incision until the cavity is reached. The lung is moved forward and caudally so that the posterior aspect of the mediastinal pleura, where the retro-esophageal space lies, is visible. A longitudinal 7-9 cm incision is done to this pleura, between the vertebral spine and the esophagus, just above the azygos vein in a cephalic direction parallel to the first two mentioned structures (Figure 1), immediately afterwards, blunt dissection with the surgeon´s index finger is done from the site of incision entering the retroesophageal space to finally reach the retropharyngeal space (Figure 2), it is obligatory to feel the previously inserted naso-gastric tube to secure and locate the esophagus so no accidental lesions occur. The majority of inferior DNM invade the mediastinum through these spaces, when performing this maneuver usually a considerable amount of purulent exudate is seen.

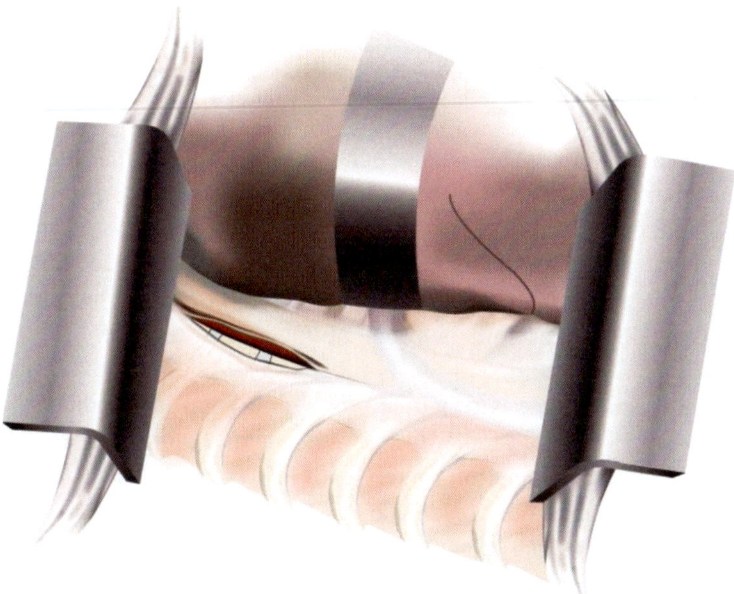

Figure 1. Incision of the posterior mediastinum between the esophagus and vertebral bodies in order to reach the retro-esophageal space. (Reproduced with permission). [26].

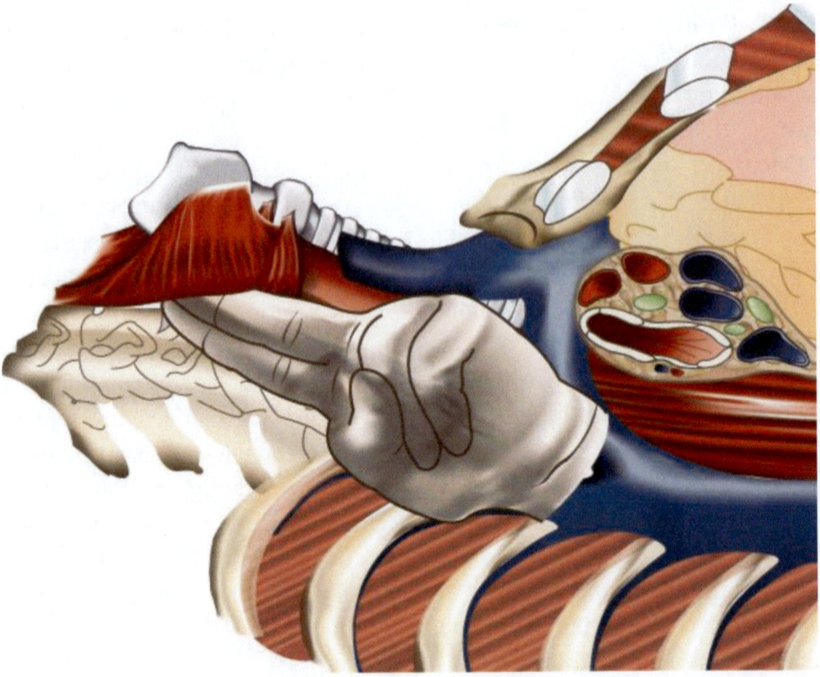

Figure 2. Once the retro-esophageal space is opened, blunt dissection in a cephalic direction is made to reach the retropharyngeal space, achieving complete drainage of the posterior mediastinum. (Reproduced with permission) [26].

Next, to drain the visceral zone a logitudinal 6 cm incision is also made in the mediastinal pleura parallel to the superior vena cava (Figure 3), once this is achieved, gentle blunt dissection is done within the great vessels and major airways, opening the pre-tracheal fascia assuring a uniform space not limited by exudative loculations or independent cavities; it is rare to find exudate in this zone but independent from the origin of infection, it must be dissected and drained.

The pre-vascular zone is penetrated through a 7 cm longitudinal incision to the mediastinal pleura, parallel to the right internal thoracic artery (Figure 4), dissecting and advancing the fingers with their anterior face towards both mammary arteries until they reach the contralateral cavity and opening the corresponding mediastinal pleura to drain the left thoracic cavity; also redirection of the fingers towards the suprasternal notch is performed until the pre-tracheal space is reached. Exudate may drain from this maneuver, especially from infections originated in the anterior neck or thorax.

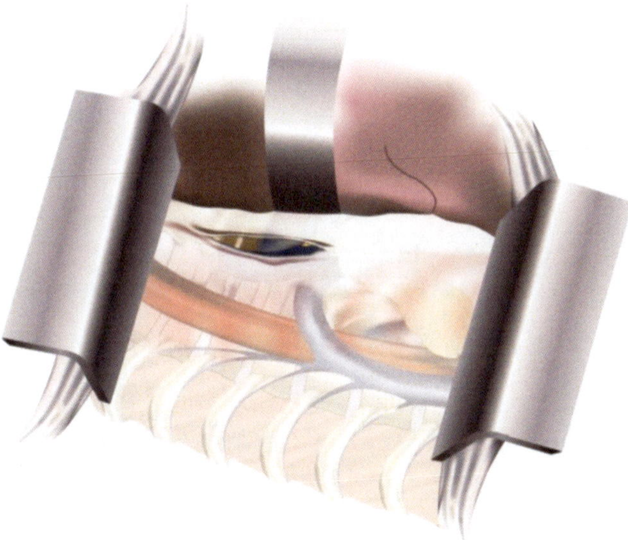

Figure 3. Incision performed to reach de visceral zone parallel to the superior vena cava. (Reproduced with permission). [26].

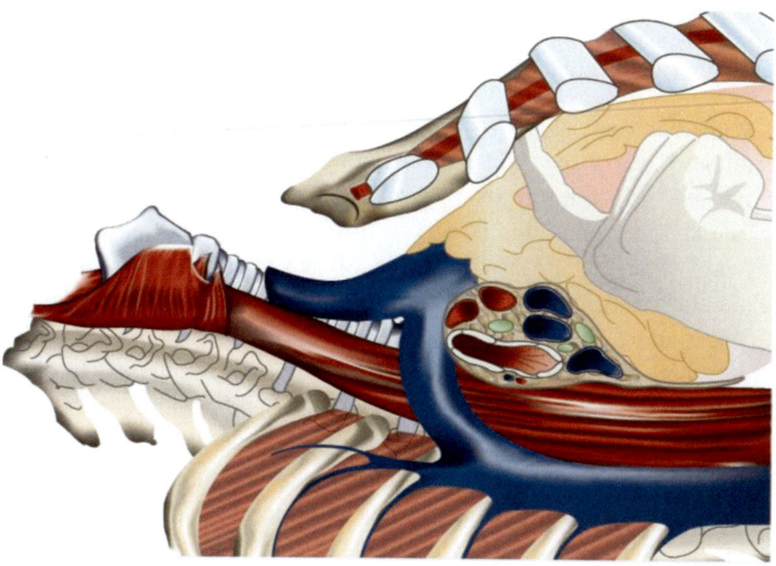

Figure 4. Site of entry to the anterior mediastinum to communicate the right thoracic cavity, pre-tracheal space and contralateral thoracic cavity. (Reproduced with permission). [26].

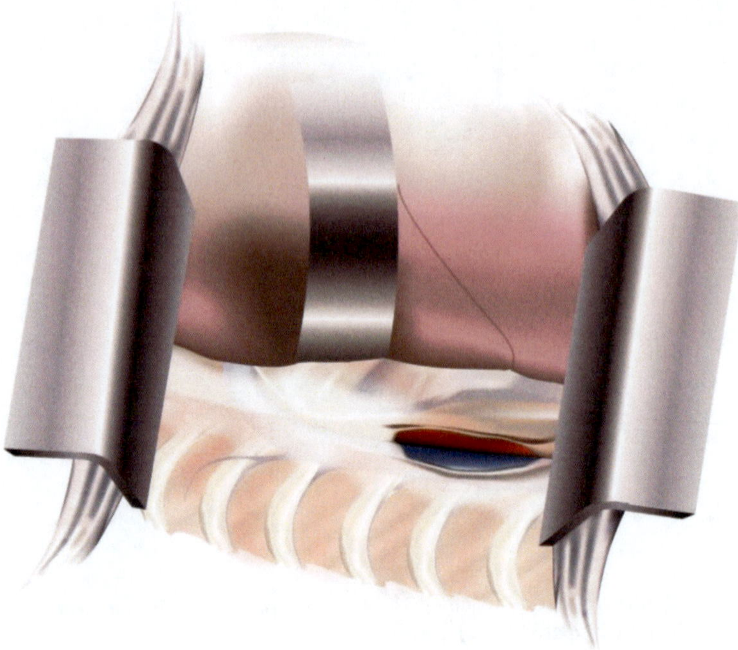

Figure 5. Incision of posterior and inferior mediastinum between the azygos vein and the esophagus. (Reproduced with permission). [26].

A fourth 9 cm incision is made to the right mediastinal pleura beginning one centimeter below the right inferior pulmonary vein caudally towards the diaphragm between the azygos vein and the esophagus (Figure 5) into the retro-visceral zone, once this is accomplished, blunt dissection is continued (identifying again the naso-gastric tube) advancing until reaching the contralateral mediastinal pleura which is opened to enter the left thoracic cavity, this is addressed with the fingers placed between the azygos vein on the palmar side and the esophagus on the dorsal side, when in the left thorax, the surgeon should be able to almost surround the descending aorta on its anterior and lateral aspects (Figure 6).

When all these maneuvers are performed correctly all mediastinal zones have been drained correctly, the next step is to perform lavage of the cavity and all opened spaces with copious amounts of sterile solution until crystalline water is seen upon suction; two chest tubes (28 – 32 Fr) are placed from independent incisions entering just above the diaphragmatic insertion, one directed to the apical and posterior side of the cavity to drain mostly fluid and the other towards the anterior and superior cavity to drain fluid and air.

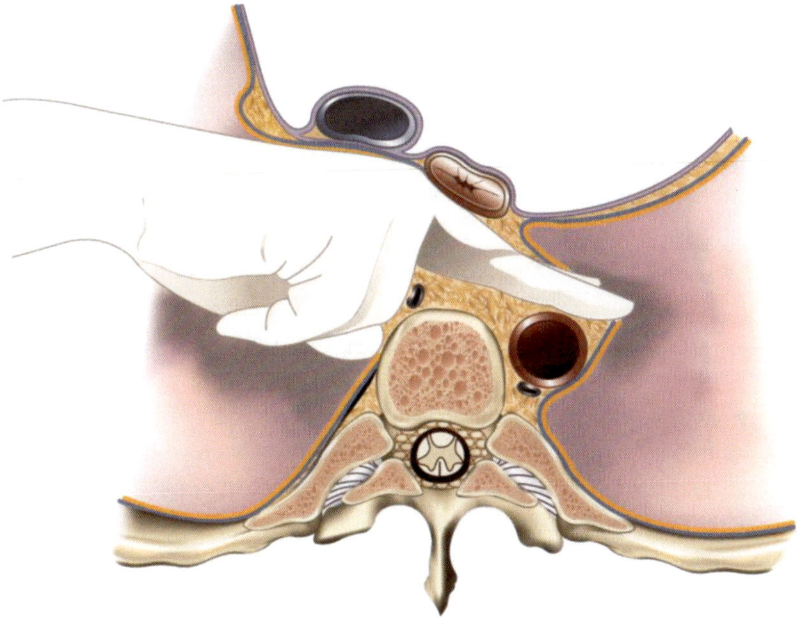

Figure 6. Passage of the surgeon´s fingers from the right to the left thoracic cavity to drain and lavage the contralateral cavity. (Reproduced with permission). [26].

The thoracotomy is closed in the usual fashion, the patient is placed in a dorsal decubitus position, unclamping of the right airway is performed so a third chest tube could be placed on the 5th left intercostal space and directed towards the posterior and superior side of the ipsilateral thoracic cavity. It is important to note that fluid cultures should be sent to investigate bacterial growth for aerobes and anaerobes so that tailored antibiotic therapy could be implemented in the post-operative period.

The right chest tubes are connected as a closed circuit (usually with a "Y" connector) to a water seal system, and the left chest tube is also placed on an independent water seal, they are usually retrieved once drainage reduces to a minimum (approximately 14 days) either with no growth on new fluid cultures (or negative gram stains) or if the fluid has a macroscopically trasudate appearance. A tracheotomy should only be considered if prolonged need for ventilator care is warranted. It is the authors´ experience that tracheotomies are usually indicated in a non-systematic way proving to make the patients more prone to post-operative pneumonias.

Misthos et al. is the only group to prospectively study the benefits of this technique when performed with a cervicotomy for DNM, where group A consisted of patients operated from a transcervical and transthoracic approach, and group B drained only though a transcervical method, after performing a multivariate analysis they concluded that a combined transthoracic and cervical debridement / drainage of the mediastinum is the only favorable factor for survival in patients with DNM (OR = 9.99, 95% CI = 1.02 - 97.49) emphasizing that less extensive approaches led to unsatisfactory results and high reoperation rates. [4]

Other Open Techniques

Many authors have also drained the mediastinum through different incisions with acceptable results; however the authors believe these have more limitations than the technique described above. Kocher et al. [9] reported 17 patients with transsternal or clamshell incisions with one fatality, Balkan et al. [10] presented a case drained by a clamshell incision due to a bilateral empyema associated with the mediastinal process. Ris et al. [11] operated three patients through the clamshell technique with one casualty; every case described had a bilateral empyema. As it has been exposed, clamshell approach conveys an ample range of exposure to attend both thoracic cavities and the mediastinum, however this is a limited surgery because reaching the retro-visceral zone is challenging, and also osteomyelitis of the sternum could arise. On the other hand, being this the largest thoracic incision, patients have a great risk for post-operative pain and prolonged mechanical ventilation with deleterious consequences.

The transsternal and/or trans-pericardial incision is a scarcely reported technique with varying grades of success, Stella et al. [12] reported one case of a patient who suffered from a left parapharyngeal abscess, treated through a transsternal and trans-pericardial surgery with an uneventful post-operative course and discharge at day 22. Núñez-Bustos et al. [13] analyzed 17 patients from which 52.9% where approached through a transsternal incision with 29.4% mortality. As it is shown, mortality with transsternal incision is comparable with the global reported mortality by other techniques, however it is worth mentioning that this is an uncomfortable exposure of the surgical field when attempting to drain the posterior zone with the added fact that sternal osteomyelitis is an imminent risk.

Bilateral thoracotomy is also an option, however as exposed in previous reports, the same result can be achieved by draining the left thoracic cavity though a right postero-lateral incision.

Subxiphoid incisions have also been reported, Guan et al. [14] proposed in their paper the use of this approach for patients that have a DNM limited to the anterior mediastinum, connecting the transcervical dissection with the subxiphoid incision by a tube, assessed with a thoracoscope, reporting a 6.7% mortality. Chen et al. [15] applied this technique in one patient in his study of 18 cases with DNM, De Freitas et al. [16] utilized it in a patient operated from a transcervical incision for placement of a mediastinal drainage with success. Wheatley et al. proposed to utilize this technique also to place a drainage system into the mediastinum since a transcervical approach is not sufficient to achieve successful results. The authors believe this is a failed attempt to do a minimally invasive surgery the wrong way because more spaces need to be addressed during mediastinal drainage and lavage.

A few number of authors describe the use of a mediastinoscope to aid in the transcervical approach, this could be an option for superior DNM facilitating dissection of the affected planes during a cervicotomy. [15, 17]

Minimally Invasive Approach

Based on the principle that DNM is a mostly purulent exudate producing disease and in very rare and isolated cases a true necrosectomy is needed, several authors have advocated the idea that a thoracoscopic approach is justified when the patient is hemodynamically stable, but not under severe septic conditions. [8, 18-20] The authors believe that this technique is eventually going to substitute a right thoracotomy for drainage and lavage of the mediastinum for several reasons; a) pain dramatically decreases when 11 mm incisions are made compared to 20-30 cm incisions, not only at skin level but the fact that no intercostal spaces are forced open, b) surgery and recovery time also is reduced achieving comparable or better results as exposed in the literature. This procedure was first described by Robberts et al. [5] in one patient but later improved and validated by various authors. [21-25] Wakahara et al. [24] also performed a minithoracotomy in 11 patients from the right side being successful in all with no mortality, also Melo et al. [22] reported three patients treated by this method without any fatality, finally Kozuki et al. [21] presented the case of a 50-year-old man that was drained by thoracoscopic surgery with an uneventful outcome; the authors agree that with this less invasive approach as an effective modality for draining the posterior mediastinum, patients will have a better prognosis when treated for this disease.

With patient placed in the left lateral decubitus position 11 mm incisions are done in the seventh intercostal space (ICS) below the scapular angle, fifth ICS in the middle axillary line, and third ICS posterior axillary line, if necessary an anterior 6 cm accessory mini-thoracotomy can be performed for ease and maneuverability during the procedure. Roberts et al. [5] made 3 incisions: in the 7th (anterior axillary line), 8th (posterior axillary line) and 9th (mid-axillary line) without the need of an accessory incision.

Once in the cavity the same spaces are searched as described for the right thoracotomy, these are incised utilizing cautery and grasping the mediastinal tissue with a ring forceps, in some occasions a red rubber catheter may be placed from the cervical spaces into the cervical incision to guide the surgeon from when working in the thoracic cavity, also the azygos vein could be stapled and divided facilitating manipulation of tissues and mediastinal drainage. The contralateral side could also be explored by thoracoscopy with placement of chest tubes in the traditional fashion.

The great results achieved with this technique urgently mandate studies with a larger sample size for assurance that future patients may receive this approach; undoubtedly video assisted surgery will substitute a right thoracotomy when minimally invasive surgery gains terrain within general thoracic surgeons.

Cervicotomy

As described in chapter 2 the cervical region is approached though an incision that goes along with the sternocleidomastoid muscle allowing entrance to the cervical spaces, with the option of extending it medially so that a transcervical dissection could be performed. It has not been clarified if this should be done before or after the thoracic incision, however it is the author´s opinion that it is better to do it before because of the extensive debridement that could potentially lead to more purulent exudate within the mediastinal spaces allowing the surgeon to adequately drain when in the thorax.

Conclusion

Drainage of the mediastinal spaces in DNM has been a very discussed subject, however it is the authors´ suggestion that all patients with a limited superior DNM, only a cervicotomy be performed when no other risk factors for mortality are present; if the infectious process has reached below the tracheal carina, the procedure of choice is a right thoracotomy in centers without experience in minimally invasive surgeries, but when video assisted thoracoscopic surgery is a regular practice, this should be the method of choice.

References

[1] Pearse HE. Mediastinitis following cervical suppuration. *Ann Surg* 1938;108:580.

[2] Endo S, Murayama F, Hasegawa T, Yamamoto S, Yamaguchi T, Sohara Y, Fuse K, Miyata M, Nishino H. Guideline of surgical management based on diffusion of descending necrotizing mediastinitis. *Jpn J Thorac Cardiovasc Surg* 1999;47(1):14-19.

[3] Dajer-Fadel W, Ibarra-Pérez C, Solís-Suarez J, Sánchez-Velázquez L, Tortolero-Sánchez C, Borrego-Borrego R, Navarro-Reynoso F, Argüero-Sánchez R. Superior and Inferior Descending Necrotizing Mediastinitis, 100 cases. *Chest* 2013;144:117A-117A.

[4] Misthos P, Katsaragakis S, Kakaris S, Theodorou D, Skottis I. Descending necrotizing anterior mediastinitis: analysis of survival and surgical treatment modalities. *J Oral Maxillofac Surg* 2007;65(4):635-639.

[5] Roberts JR, Smythe WR, Weber RW, Lanutti M, Rosengard BR, Kaiser LR. Thoracoscopic management of descending necrotizing mediastinitis. *Chest* 1997;112(3):850-854.

[6] Inoue Y, Gika M, Nozawa K, Ikeda Y, Takanami I. Optimum drainage method in descending necrotizing mediastinitis. *Interact Cardiovasc Thorac Surg* 2005;4:189–192.

[7] Iwata T, Sekine Y, Shibuya K, et al. Early open thoracotomy and mediastinopleural irrigation for severe descending necrotizing mediastinitis. *Eur. J. Cardiothorac Surg* 2005;28:384–388.

[8] Marty-Ane CH, Alauzen M, Alric P, Serres-Cousine O, Mary H. Descending necrotizing mediastinitis. Advantage of mediastinal drainage with thoracotomy. *J Thorac Cardiovasc Surg* 1994;107:55–61.

[9] Kocher GJ, Hoksch B, Caversaccio M, Wiegand J, Schmid RA. Diffuse descending necrotizing mediastinitis: surgical therapy and outcome in a single-centre series. *Eur J Cardiothorac Surg* 2012;42(4):e66-72.

[10] Balkan ME, Oktar GL, Oktar MA. Descending necrotizing mediastinitis: a case report and review of the literature. *Int Surg* 2001;86(1):62-66.

[11] Ris HB, Banic A, Furrer M, Caversaccio M, Cerny A, Zbären P. Descending necrotizing mediastinitis: surgical treatment via clamshell approach. *Ann Thorac Surg* 1996;62(6):1650-1654.

[12] Stella F, Petrella F. Transsternal trenspericardial approach for acute descending necrotizing mediastinitis. *J Thorac Cardiovasc Surg* 2005;129(1):212-214.

[13] Núñez-Bustos CM, Ibarra-Celaya JM, Guzmán-de Alba E, Aguilar-Mena ME. Resúmenes de los trabajos libres del LXXII Congreso Nacional de Neumología y Cirugía de Tórax (Mérida 2013). *Neumol Cir Torax* 2013;72:66-115.

[14] Guan X, Zhang WJ, Liang X, Liang X, Wang F, Guo X, Zhou Y. Optimal surgical options for descending necrotizing mediastinitis of the anterior mediastinum. *Cell Biochem Biophys* 2014;70(1):109-114.

[15] Chen KC, Chen JS, Kuo SW, Huang PM, Hsu HH, Lee JM, Lee YC. Descending necrotizing mediastinitis: a 10-year surgical experience in a single institution. *J Thorac Cardiovasc Surg* 2008;136(1):191-198.

[16] Wheatley MJ, Stirling MC, Kirsh MM, Gago O, Orringer MB. Descending necrotizing mediastinitis: transcervical drainage is not enough. *Ann Thorac Surg* 1990;49(5):780-784.

[17] Ishinga H, Otsu K, Sakaida H, Miyamura T, Nakamura S, Kitano M, Tenpaku H, Takao M, Kobayashi M, Takeuchi K. Descending necrotizing mediastinitis from deep neck infection. *Eur Arch Otorhinolaryngol* 2013;270(4):1463-1466.

[18] De Freitas RP, Fahy CP, Brooker DS, et al. Descending necrotising mediastinitis: a safe treatment algorithm. *Eur Arch Otorhinolaryngol* 2007;264:181–187.

[19] Freeman RK, Vallieres E, Verrier ED, Karmy-Jones R, Wood DE. Descending necrotizing mediastinitis: an analysis of the effects of serial surgical debridement on patient mortality. *J Thorac Cardiovasc Surg* 2000;119:260–267.

[20] Min HK, Choi YS, Shim YM, Sohn YI, Kim J. Descending necrotizing mediastinitis: a minimally invasive approach using video-assisted thoracoscopic surgery. *Ann Thorac Surg* 2004;77:306–310.

[21] Kozuki A, Shinozaki H, Tajima A, Kase K. Successful treatment for descending necrotizing mediastinitis with severe thoracic emphysema using video-assited thoracoscopic surgery. *Gen Thorac Cardiovasc Surg* 2012;58(11):584-587.

[22] Melo CB, Sarmento PA, Imaeda CJ, Daud, Hashimoto FN, Leão LE. Descending necrotizing mediastinitis: minimally invasive thoracic surgical treatment. *J Bras Pneumol* 2010;36(6):812-818.
[23] Suga A, Inoue Y, Takeichi H, Yamada S, Iwazaki M. A case of an elderly patient treated for descending necrotizing mediastinitis. *Gen Thorac Cardiovasc Surg* 2011;59(9):623-626.
[24] Wakahara T, Tanaka Y, Maniwa Y, Nishio W, Yoshimura M. Successful management of descending necrotizing mediastinitis. *Asian Cardiovasc Thorac Ann* 2011;19(3-4):228-231.
[25] Hsin MK, Yim AP. Video assisted thoracoscopic surgery is a valuable approach for the management of descending necrotizing mediastinitis. *Ann Surg* 2011;253(5):1055.
[26] Dajer-Fadel WL, Ibarra-Pérez C, Argüero-Sánchez R. Mediastinal drainage in descending necrotizing mediastinitis. *Asian Cardiovasc Thorac Ann* 2013;21:493-495.

In: Mediastinal Infections
Editor: Walid Leonardo Dajer-Fadel
ISBN: 978-1-63463-369-7

Chapter 6

Medical Management for Descending Necrotizing Mediastinitis

***J. D. Casillas-Enriquez*[1,*] *and W. L. Dajer-Fadel*[2]**
[1]Pneumology Department, Pachuca General Hospital, Pachuca, Hidalgo, Mexico
[2]Cardiothoracic Surgery Department, General Hospital of Mexico "Dr. Eduardo Liceaga", Mexico City, Mexico

Abstract

Descending necrotizing mediastinitis (DNM) produces an overwhelming inflammatory response in susceptible patients, it is well known that the standard of care corresponds to surgical treatment to drain and lavage the mediastinal areas and fascia, however, medical management stands as the backbone in caring for these patients; many evidence based antibiotic regimens have been proposed in the past, they are based on the primary pathogens culprit for this illness, which include aerobe and anaerobe bacteria as the main producers of DNM, for which a directed therapy has to be implemented in every patient. Also, new therapies are emerging for adjuvant care, the main ones are hyperbaric oxygen, plasmapheresis, and fluoroscopic percutaneous drainage; these

* Correspondence to: José Domingo Casillas Enriquez, Email address: jdcasienri@hotmail.com.

have proven to be helpful, however more randomized controlled trials may have to be performed to validate their use. Septic patients such as these are being rapidly identified throughout concentration hospitals with better results being constantly sought. There are many surgical and clinical efforts that need to be done when treating DNM; definitely, this is a cooperative task among specialties as a multidisciplinary approach that many times has proven to obtain the best results.

Introduction

Mediastinitis can be divided into acute and chronic, usually both are of infectious etiology, and the first is generally related to bacterial infections, whilst the latter, to granulomatous or fibrous processes [1]. The acute type is a severe infection and inflammatory process of the connective tissues that comprises the inter-pleural mediastinic space surrounding the middle thoracic viscera. [2, 3] DNM is one of the most lethal and severe forms of infection for which no medical treatment alone has ever been successful, this has been proven since the work of Pierce et al. who reported 110 patients with a mortality reduction from 86% to 35% between the ones that were not drained and the group that underwent surgical drainage and lavage [4]. Even with the most advanced antibiotic, surgical, anesthetic and ICU treatment protocols, DNM continues to be a condition with high mortality (40%) and life threatening complications [5, 6, 7]. Continued work and effort is done to raise clinicians´ awareness towards this dreadful underestimated disease. In this chapter we present a description of the medical treatment based on antibiotic protocols, also, a brief review of novel therapies that might change the course of this pathologic process.

Antibiotics

DNM management consists in directing the appropriate antibiotic therapy against all the possible pathogens. The increased incidence in anaerobial bacteria within the mediastinum has taken a greater appraisal of their role in this disease, and the re-evaluation on this condition´s correct choice of antibiotics [8]. The most frequent microorganisms are β-hemolytic *Streptococcus* (71.5%) and mixed anaerobic flora (27.8%), which provoke small vessel thrombosis that favor growth of these type of bacteria such as

Prevotella, Porphyromonas spp., Fusobacterium spp. and Peptostreptococcus spp [9]. There are also few reports about the involvement of Bacterioides fragilis. When faced with a clinical-radiological suspicion of DNM, empirical antibiotic therapy is justified. Such conduct must be efficacious against anaerobic and aerobic flora. Ideally beginning with a double antibiotic scheme conformed by third generation cephalosporins (ceftriaxone) and clindamycin or metronidazole while waiting for culture reports and acting upon them, modifying treatment if necessary, remembering that no growth on culture is positive in 20% of the time [8, 9].

There are also other available options: a) carbapenems (imipenem cilastatin or meropenem) plus clindamycin, b) fourth generation cephalosporins (cefepime) plus clindamycin, c) penicillin combinations (amoxicillin, ticarcillin or piperacillin) and a β-lactamase inhibitor (clavulanic acid, sulbactam or tazobactam) plus clindamycin which are adequate for anaerobes, enterobacteriae and *Staphylococcus aureus*.

In case of developing a methicillin resistant *Staphylococcus aureus* strain, adding vancomycin or linezolid to the therapy is suggested.

Full dose systemic antibacterial therapy should be given for at least 4 – 6 weeks, and adjusting it in cases of renal or hepatic failure [10, 11]. Even more, co-infection and/or sole isolation of fungal agents is still controversial. Ridder et al. [8]. reported two patients where a fungal origin was grown, however, antifungal treatment was not utilized, since these patients were not immunocompromised and the presence of Candida spp. was considered a result of contamination within the pharyngeal wall; taking this into account, the authors do not recommend treatment for these microbes unless a quantitative colony count exceeds 100,000.

Monitoring and Medical Support

MND is by definition a septic process due to a secondary inflammatory systemic infection. This process could evolve into a severe form, complicated by an acute organic dysfunction followed by septic shock, producing tissue hypo-perfusion, manifested as hypertension refractory to fluid resuscitation and presence of elevated serum lactate [12]. Initial management should be based on the last edition of the Surviving Sepsis Campaign Guidelines (2013), the two most important points of the guide are organized in two care "packages": an initial management within the first six hours, and a second, instituted at the ICU [13]. Better results are seen when treatment is performed based on these conducts [14].

Initial treatment principles are to deliver cardiorespiratory resuscitation and mitigating immediate threats of uncontrolled infection. Strong recommendations include fluid resuscitation with the exact required components such as, selection and quantity of solutions, type and intensity of the appropriate hemodynamic monitoring, and the role of adjuvant vasoactive agents; these are all still subject of debate. However, fluid control is considered essential, it is crucial to apply a standardized treatment protocol in a fast and effective manner to reach the following goals: [13]

1. Maintain a central venous pressure of 8 mmHg
2. Maintain a mean arterial pressure >65 mmHg
3. A urine output >0.5 ml/kg/h.
4. Central venous oxygen saturation >70% or a mixed saturation >65%.

This should be accomplished in the first six hours; once in the ICU, if signs of tissue hypoperfusion persist, dobutamine infusion should begin at a maximum of 20 mcg/Kg/min, or blood transfusions to achieve an erythrocyte count of ≥30%. If refractory hypotension persists despite the previous measures, consider infusion of IV vasopressors (ideally norepinephrine), oxygen therapy and mechanical ventilation, according to the patient´s needs [15]. Empiric treatment should be ideally started during the first hour after a diagnosis of sepsis is done, culture samples are taken before or at the beginning of disease, this regimen should be started as soon as possible; a delay in applying these measures, is associated to a higher mortality [16].

After the first six hours, the patient should be exchanged to an ICU ward because care should have a close follow-up, vital organ support and complication avoidance, all this after a surgical intervention for DNM, which in this case is essential and has a direct impact on survival [8, 9].

Treating Complications

In general, a mean of 74% of post-operative complications are seen in patients with DNM, from which septic shock is the most common and severe in 23.3-50% of the cases [8, 17]. Ridder et al. reported 40 (88.9%) survivors, with a mean hospital LOS of 36.3 days (range 9 – 139 days), 71.1% where treated at the ICU during a mean of 11.7 days, 73.3% had more than one surgery under general anesthesia for the drainage and debridement of the involved spaces, the three most common complications were pleural effusion (72%), pneumonia (42%) and severe sepsis or septic shock (35%); [8] Also fistulas have been reported as common complication [18].

The advantage of granulated sugar over infected tissues to destroy bacteria has been utilized in open wound care of infected sternotomies with good results, unfortunately this only works at a regional level [19]. Nowadays, the use of negative pressure wound therapy for the treatment of infected wounds, based on microporous polyurethane sponges that are placed and covered by a plastic material which is cut in the middle where a suctioning device is connected, producing a continuous negative pull on the tissues adjacent to the sponges, promotes neovascularization and leukocyte migration to the affected area [20]. This therapy has been mostly described for sternal dehiscence and post-operative mediastinitis, which is the type of infection generally seen in cardiac surgeries and will be discussed in the following chapters.

New Therapies

The use of hyperbaric chamber oxygen therapy is a proposed adjuvant treatment for the care of these patients, however randomized controlled trials (RCT) are needed to evaluate its results, in the first experimental studies Vedat et al. reported a significant ($p = <0.05$) reduction in the bacterial count of patients that received such therapy adjunct to antibiotics compared to the ones that only received one or the other alone; they also compared other therapies such as teicoplanine or vancomyacin with hyperbaric oxygen (HO) and none where significantly different from the use of linezolid and HO. They concluded that the efficacy of HO therapy is similar when combined with vancomyacin, teicoplanine and linezolid, and that the combined treatment of HO with antibiotics produces a synergistic effect. Ridder et al., during his study, delivered this treatment to six of his patients improving their symptoms [8, 20, 21]. This therapy has the sufficient experimental background to be applied in RCT and prove its efficacy in DNM.

Plasmapheresis is a therapeutic technique that eliminates by convective transport through a semipermeable membrane high molecular weight substances from plasma such as auto-antibodies, immune complexes, light chains, endotoxins, cryoglobulins and lypoproteins. When using fresh frozen plasma as replacement fluid, the consumed plasmatic factors are substituted; therefore, opsonization capacity is restored improving coagulation abnormalities, both present in sepsis (Figure 1) [22, 23]. This therapy has historically played an important role in the treatment of sepsis to modulate the overwhelming systemic inflammatory response of these patients. Schmidt et al. performed an observational pilot study examining the effects of this technique in patients exposed to surgery for the treatment of a septic process, where they accomplished a 28% mortality reduction [24]. Steygmar et al. found that endotoxins and interleukin 6 produced by bacteria are eliminated through plasma exchange therapy; also Gardlund et al. took samples of interleukin 1β and tumor necrosis factor α finding a descent in the latter with this therapy. Finally McClelland et al. demonstrated that endotoxins, tumor necrosis factor and immunosuppressive prostaglandins are cleansed; however, endotoxin is the only marker that can be measured before a plasmapheresis procedure is performed [25, 26, 27].

Since 1979 various reports have been published regarding plasmapheresis in septic patients, however they are only brief communications or with a small sample size without being properly studied in a clinical trial. Busund et al. proved that this is a safe procedure in the treatment of septic patients with an absolute mortality risk reduction of 20.5%, concluding that plasmapheresis can be an important adjuvant to conventional treatment in patients with sepsis and septic shock, nonetheless, this option has not yet been accepted as the standard of care [28, 23].

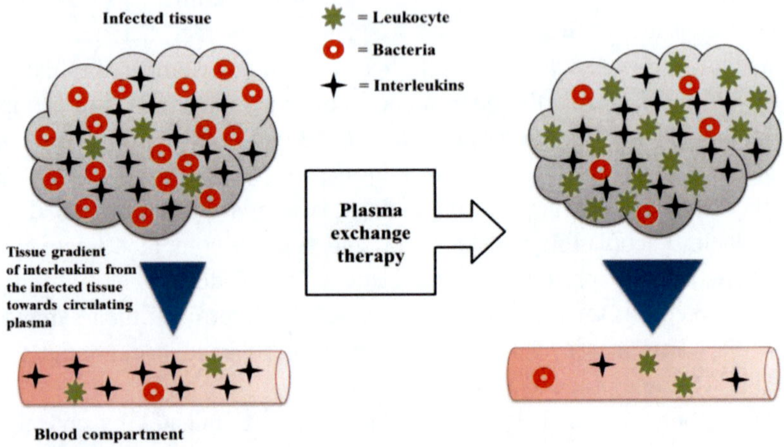

Figure 1. Schematic representation of how plasmapheresis reduces bacteria concentration of the infected tissue stimulating migration by concentration gradients of interleukins, bacteria and leukocytes from the septic foci to the vascular space which is subject to cleansing by this therapy.

Based on what has been exposed above and backed-up by literature, the next step is to demonstrate its benefit and reproducibility in patients with mediastinitis. The only authors that have thoroughly studied this is a Russian group that decreased mortality from 35.3% to 12.5% by using this method, they applied this therapy for patients with mediastinitis from any etiology. With these uplifting results, the use of plasmapheresis should be trialed for DNM in the near future [29, 30].

Another therapy with satisfactory results is the use of guided catheters. This is justified by the authors by emphasizing the fact that necrotic tissue in the affected spaces is small, and that the goal of surgical intervention is drainage rather than debridement. Based on this principle they compared a group of 11 patients operated the conventional way with 20 patients treated by a 7-French catheter, originally fabricated for percutaneous transhepatic cholangio drainage [PTCD kit, Create Medic] placing it under fluoroscopic and ultrasonographic guidance into the infected spaces. Both groups were compared for mortality (with 0% in both groups), ICU LOS, changes in C-reactive protein levels, duration of antibiotic therapy, and duration of mechanical ventilation, all of which were not significantly different; however: secondary wound infection, growth of resistant bacteria, number of days before oral feeding, and use of plasma infusion / analgesics, were less seen in the percutaneous group [31]. Unfortunately this is the only report utilizing this technique worthy of mentioning, and surely requires more attention for future trials to gain worldwide acceptance.

Conclusion

When recognized late or treated inadequately, DNM is an infection with high mortality, this is why if suspicion of this disease is imminent, early diagnosis and use of wide spectrum antibiotics with adequate surgical drainage and lavage have a great impact on survival. It needs to be treated as a medical emergency, independently of the surgical approach (which is obligatory), a directed antibiotic therapy has to be sought. Future investigations not only have to be focused towards quick identification of pathogenic agents and development of new antibiotics, but also new adjunct therapies such as hyperbaric oxygen, plasmapheresis or percutaneous drainages that could change the course of the systemic inflammatory response and favor a less severe organic dysfunction, to improve prognosis in this highly mortal disease.

References

[1] Athanassiadi KA. Infections of the mediastinum. *Thorac Surg Clin* 2009;19:37-45.

[2] Sancho LM, Minamoto H, Fernandez A, Sennes LU, Jatene FB. Descending necrotizing mediastinitis: a retrospective surgical experience. *Eur J Cardiothorac Surg* 1999;16:200–205.

[3] Mihos P, Potaris K, Gakidis I, Papadakis D, Rallis G. Management of descending necrotizing mediastinitis. *J Oral Maxillofac Surg* 2004;62:966–972.

[4] Pearse HE. Mediastinitis following cervical suppuration. *Ann Surg* 1938;108:580-611.

[5] Singhal P, Kejriwal N, Lin Z, Tsutsui R, Ullal R. Optimal surgical management of descending necrotising mediastinitis: our experience and review of literature. *Heart Lung Circ* 2008;17:124 –128.

[6] Misthos P, Katsaragakis S, Kakaris S, Theodorou D, Skottis I. Descending necrotizing anterior mediastinitis: analysis of survival and surgical treatment modalities. *J Oral Maxillofac Surg* 2007;65:635–639.

[7] Urschel Jr HC, Patel AN, Razzuk MA, Hoover SJ, Razzuk LM, Montano R. Chronic mediastinitis. In: Patterson GA, Cooper JD, Deaslauriers J, Lerut AE. MR, Luketich JD, Rice TW. Pearson's thoracic and esophageal surgery. Vol I. 3rd ed. Philadelphia: Churchill Livingstone; 2008. p. 1529-1536.

[8] Ridder GJ, Maier W, Kinzer S, Teszler C, Boedeker C, Pfeiffer J. Descending necrotizing mediastinitis. Conttemporary trends in etiology, diagnosis, management and outcome. *Ann Surg* 2010;251:528-534.

[9] Deu-Martín M, Saez-Barba M, López-Sanz I, Alcaraz-Peñarrocha R, Romero-Vielva L, Solé-Montserrat J. Factores de riesgo de mortalidad en la mediastinitis necrosante descendente. *Arch Bronconeumol* 2010; 46:182-187.

[10] Murray PM, Finegold SM. Anaerobic mediastinitis. *Rev Infect Dis* 1984;6:S123-127.

[11] Brook I, Frazier EH. Microbiology of mediastinitis. *Arch Intern Med* 1996;12;156:333-336.

[12] Levy MM, Fink MP, Marshall JC, et al. 2001 SCCM/ESICM /ACCP/ATS/SIS International Sepsis Definitions Conference. *Crit Care Med* 2003;31:1250-1256.

[13] Dellinger RP, Levy MM, Rhodes A, , Annane D, Gerlach H, Opal SM, Sevransky JE, Sprung CL, Douglas IS, Jaeschke R, Osborn TM,

Nunnally ME, Townsend SR, Reinhart K, Kleinpell RM, Angus DC, Deutschman CS, Machado FR, Rubenfeld GD, Webb SA, Beale RJ, Vincent JL, Moreno R. Surviving Sepsis Campaign: international guidelines for management of severe sepsis and septic shock: 2012. *Crit Care Med* 2013;41:580-637.

[14] Ferrer R, Artigas A, Levy MM, Blanco J, González-Díaz G, Garnacho-Montero J, Ibáñez J, Palencia E, Quintana M, de la Torre-Prados MV. Improvement in process of care and outcome after a multicenter severe sepsis educational program in Spain. *JAMA* 2008; 299:2294-2303.

[15] Levy MM, Dellinger RP, Townsend SR, Linde-Zwirble WT, Marshall JC, Bion J, Schorr C, Artigas A, Ramsay G, Beale R, Parker MM, Gerlach H, Reinhart K, Silva E, Harvey M, Regan S, Angus DC. The Surviving Sepsis Campaign: results of an international guideline-based performance improvement program targeting severe sepsis. *Crit Care Med* 2010;38:367-374.

[16] Paul M, Shani V, Muchtar E, Kariv G, Robenshtok E, Leibovici L. Systematic re- view and meta-analysis of the efficacy of appropriate empiric antibiotic therapy for sepsis. *Antimicrob Agents Chemother* 2010; 54:4851-4863.

[17] Dajer-Fadel WL, Ibarra-Pérez C, Solís-Suárez JA, Sánchez-Velázquez LD, Tortolero-Sánchez C, Borrego-Borrego R, Navarro-Reynoso FP, Argüero-Sánchez, R. Superior and inferior descending necrotizing mediastinitis, 100 cases. *Chest* 2013;144,117A-117A.

[18] Dajer-Fadel WL, Ibarra-Pérez C, Sánchez-Velazquez LD, Borrego-Borrego R, Navarro-Reynoso FP, Argüero-Sánchez R. Descending necrotizing mediastinitis below the tracheal carina. *Asian Cardiovasc Thorac Ann* 2014;22(2):176-182.

[19] De Feo M, Gregorio R, Renzulli A, Ismeno G, Romano GP, Cotrufo M. Treatment of recurrent postoperative mediastinitis with granulated sugar. *J Cardiovasc Surg* (Torino) 2000;41:715-719.

[20] Sjogren J, Gustafsson R, Nilsson J, Malmsjo M, Ingemansson R. Clinical outcome after poststernotomy mediastinitis: vacuum-assisted closure versus conventional treatment. *Ann Thorac Surg* 2005;79: 2049-2055.

[21] Vedat Turhan, M.D., Suzan Sacar, M.D., et al. Hyperbaric Oxygen as Adjunctive Therapy in Experimental Mediastinitis. *J of Surg Research* 2009;155:111–115.

[22] Mader JT, Brown GL, Guckian JC, et al. A mechanism for the amelioration by hyperbaric oxygen of experimental staphylococcal osteomyelitis in rabbits. *J Infect Dis* 1980;142:915.

[23] Rimmlé T, Kellum JA. Clinical review: Blood purification for sepsis. *Critical Care* 2011;15:205-215.

[24] Schmidt J, Mann S, Mohr VD, Lampert R, Firla U, Zirngibl H. Plasmapheresis combined with continuous venovenous hemofiltration in surgical patients with sepsis. *Intensive Care Med* 2000;26:532-537.

[25] Stegmayr BG. Plasmapheresis in severe sepsis or septic shock. *Blood Purif* 1996;14:94-101.

[26] Gardlund B, Sjölin J, Nilsson A, Roll M, Wickerts CJ, Wretlind B. Plasma levels of cytokines in primary septic shock in humans: correlation with disease severity. *J Infect Dis* 1995;172:296-301.

[27] McClelland P, Williams PS, Yaqoob M, Mostafa SM, Bone M. Multiple organ failure – a role for plasma exchange? *Intensive Care Med* 1990; 16:100-103.

[28] Busund R, Koukline V, Utrobin U, Nedashkovsky E. Plasmapheresis in severe sepsis and septic shock: a prospective, randomised, controlled trial. *Intensive Care Med* 2002;28:1434-1439.

[29] Reï SI, Aleksandrova IV, Khvatov VB, Bulava GV, Godkov MA, Borovkova NV, Fedorova NV, Abakumov MM. Immunological aspects of the early application of extracorporeal hemocorrection techniques in the complex therapy of purulent mediastinitis. *Anesteziol Reanimatol* 2008;3:38-42.

[30] Abakumov MM, Aleksandrova IV, Reï SI, Dorfman AG, Nikitina OV, Davydov BV, Matveev SB, Vasina NV. Early application of plasmapheresis for complex treatment of purulent mediastinitis. *Khirurgiia* (Mosk) 2008;2:4-9.

[31] Nakamori Y, Fujimi S, Ogura H, Kuwagata Y, Tanaka H, Shimazu T, Ueda T, Sugimoto H. Conventional open surgery versus percutaneous catheter drainage in the treatment of cervical necrotizing fasciitis and descending necrotizing mediastinitis. *AJR* 2004;182:1443-1449.

In: Mediastinal Infections
Editor: Walid Leonardo Dajer-Fadel
ISBN: 978-1-63463-369-7

Chapter 7

Ascending Necrotizing Mediastinitis

***R. Borrego-Borrego*[1,2*] *and W. L. Dajer-Fadel*[3]**
[1]Administrative Department,
Dr. Rafael Barba Ocampo Hospital (ISSSTE), Cuautla, Morelos, Mexico
[2]Thoracic Surgery Department, Angeles Acoxpa Hospital,
Mexico City, Mexico
[3]Cardiothoracic Surgery Department, General Hospital of Mexico
"Dr. Eduardo Liceaga", Mexico City, Mexico

Abstract

Rupture of sub-diaphragmatic abdominal or retroperitoneal abscesses that result in thoracic infections have been reported by several investigators. Stomach or colonic lesions have been found to be more common in the postoperative period, also duodenal and caecal ruptures have been described. When an abscess opens to the peritoneal cavity, surgical treatment by drainage and lavage of viscous, purulent exudate is in most instances enough to control the infectious process. However, quite often this complication could be fatal. If an early diagnosis is not made, severe sepsis develops in such patients. Sometimes it persists as seen in many bizarre examples, which are difficult to detect and diagnose, leading to further complications by opening into the thoracic cavity,

* Correspondence to: Rafael Borrego-Borrego, E-mail address: tofoborrego@terra.com.mx.

mediastinum and pericardium. Extension or propagation of the infectious process could begin from the kidneys, suprarenal glands, urinary tract, pancreas, retroperitoneal muscles or pelvis, disseminating by means of the lymphatic vessels, in the blood stream, or by direct invasion of retroperitoneal compartments and their fascia through adjacent tissues. When an infection with these characteristics affects the mediastinum, it causes sepsis, tissue destruction, an acute inflammatory response, or death due to multi-organic failure if not treated in a timely and appropriate manner. This is why treatment protocols should be conformed and executed by a multidisciplinary team of physicians involved in the management of the metabolic aspects of disease (electrolyte imbalances, septic shock and acute inflammatory response) at the intensive care unit and during anesthesia. The abdominal septic origin has to be attended by a general surgeon in conjunction with the cardiothoracic surgery team. In the chapter, a thorough review of the scarce literature available on the subject is presented to understand where the specialist stands when confronting this rare situation.

Introduction

According to the etiologic classification of mediastinitis there must be a differentiation, leaving as a separate chapter post-operative mediastinitis, descending necrotizing mediastinitis, mediastinitis secondary to esophageal perforation, traumatic mediastinitis and in particular ascending necrotizing mediastinitis. [1-4] Each of these pathologies have a different etiology with special features regarding treatment, evolution and prognosis.

Ascending necrotizing mediastinitis can occur as a complication of abdominal or retroperitoneal infections that spread to the mediastinum through lymphatic vessels, blood flow or diaphragmatic-peritoneum permeability, including diaphragmatic hiatuses. [3, 5-7]

Several diseases produce ascending necrotizing mediastinitis such as appendicitis, intestinal perforation, peritonitis, pyocholecyst, kidney or urinary tract infections and pancreatitis, among others. [3, 7-11]. In cases where there are two or more compartments with septic problems, they always require a complex multidisciplinary approach with sound knowledge of the overwhelming infection and systemic inflammatory response. [2, 4, 12, 13]

Principles of Infection

Peritoneal and pleural mesothelium have the same embryologic origin; mesenchymal cells migrate from the endoderm to the celomic cavity, in such a way that when they separate during fetal growth, the diaphragm will separate the abdominal from the thoracic cavities. Simultaneously, development of the mediastinal spaces begins, hiatuses are formed, and they allow abdominal structures to pass to the chest, such as the inferior vena cava, thoracic duct, esophagus and aorta. [2, 6, 7, 14]

In addition to the physiological and anatomical characteristics, there are alterations of the diaphragm which include different types of hiatal and diaphragm hernias, which if complicated, may trigger a mediastinal septic process. [14]

The diaphragm has a great amount of lymphatic and capillary vessels that constantly absorb and circulate peritoneal fluid close it, making this, one of the most important principles of infectious invasion to the mediastinum. [2,7,14]

Respiratory movement makes peritoneal fluid migrate from different abdominal regions to the sub-diaphragmatic space, in such a way that when there is a septic process of the cavity, it takes from 3 to 8 hours to spread, depending on the amount and viscosity of the material, hydrostatic pressure, oncotic pressure, breathing movements (from the negative intra-thoracic pressure) and gravity. [2,3,14-17].

The retro-peritoneum can be defined as a virtual space bounded in its superior portion by both hemi-diaphragms, inferiorly by the pelvic sub-peritoneal space, posteriorly by the transversalis fascia and anteriorly by the posterior region of the parietal peritoneum. It contains the anterior para-renal compartment, located in front of Gerota's fascia (or anterior renal fascia). It also encompasses the renal, peri-renal or posterior para-renal (located behind the posterior renal or Zuckercandl´s fascia) compartments, and finally, the area of the psoas and great vessels. [2,4,7,18,19]

The anterior para-renal compartment contains the pancreas, second and third duodenal portion, and ascending and descending colon. [4,8,18,19]

In the posterior para-renal compartment there are lymphatic nodes and adipose tissue, whilst the renal compartment contains the kidneys and the adrenal glands. [3,8,14]

The importance of knowing the retroperitoneal anatomy and viscera located in each of its compartments is to adequately categorize and determine the pathologies that affect each of these areas, and which region is important to follow up to avoid complications or fatalities. [14]

The peri-renal space is a retroperitoneal space limited by the anterior renal fascia (Gerota) and subsequently by the posterior renal fascia (Zuckercandl). These two, merge laterally to form the lateral-conal fascia. They are attached above to the diaphragmatic fascia, they are merged on top and below the adrenal gland with the iliac fascia. They define a space in the form of an inverted cone that has its origin from the embryonic migration of kidneys´ to the pelvic region until it reaches its final retroperitoneal position. [3, 14]

Overview

The first description of mediastinitis was made by Hermman Boerhaave in 1724 when in a detailed text of 70 pages he stated the clinical case of the Baron Von Vassenaer, who suffered a post-emetic perforation of the esophagus. There are multiple causes of mediastinitis divided into acute and chronic. The acute type could be post-operative, cervical descending necrotizing, after esophageal injury and of infradiaphragmatic origin. The chronic type is divided in granulomatous and fibrosing. Necrotizing ascending mediastinitis corresponds to an infradiaphragmatic septic process that invades superior fascia until it reaches any of the mediastinal zones of Shields. [2,4,9,12,20]

The ones that have a subdiaphragmatic origin can be divided into peritoneal and retroperitoneal infections. This disease extends through the peritoneal serous and retroperitoneal fascia into mediastinal spaces. It is imperative to have anatomical and embryonic knowledge of the thoracic and abdominal elements´ development in order to understand the mechanism of the disease, and select the optimal surgical approach (Figure 1). [2,3,9,12-14]

There are just a few published cases of retroperitoneal propagation which include pancreatic abscesses, and kidney / urinary tract infections. They are superposed infections that spread through the fascia, similar to what happens in the descending type, but in this case, it follows an ascending pattern which is determined by the thoracic negative pressure and respiratory movements. [3,10,11,21-23]

Peritoneal fluid circulation is responsible for the dissemination of septic intraperitoneal infections, this could propagate by contiguity to the pleura generating empyema and potentially ascending mediastinitis (Figure 2).

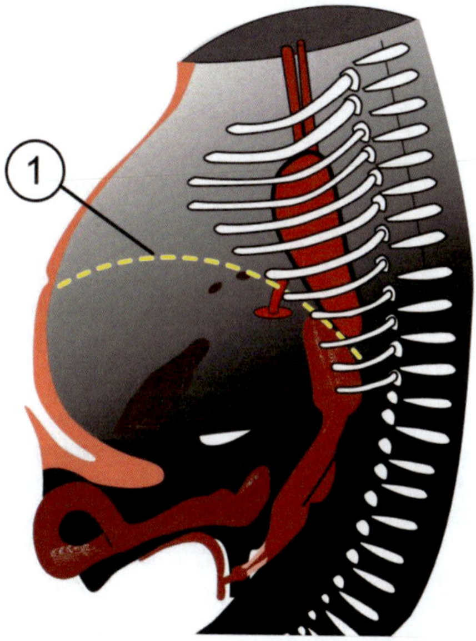

Figure 1. Celomic cavity and its interaction during embryonic development, separated by the diaphragm (number 1) to form the abdominal and thoracic cavities.

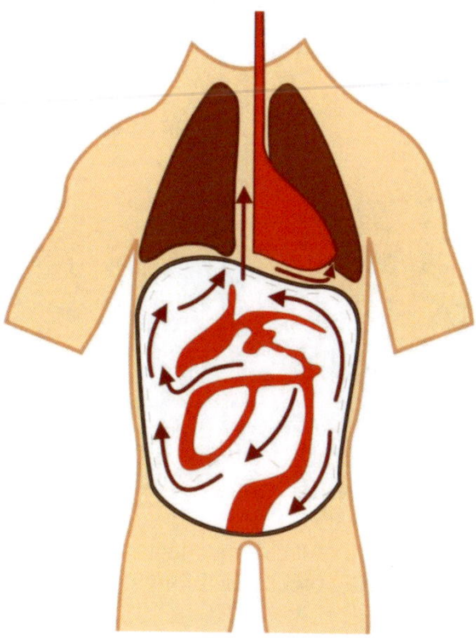

Figure 2. Peritoneal fluid circulation and its relationship to the mediastinum during a septic processes.

It can also be produced in a direct pattern due to the diaphragm´s permeability through microscopic pores in the thoracic portion of the abdomen on fibromuscular or vascular fascia and by lymphatic vessels. [3,10,11,14,22,23] Superimposed infections are defined by the ones that involve two or three anatomical compartments which could include the peritoneum, retroperitoneum, pleura and mediastinum (Figure 3). [3,7] Among the post-operative complications that could lead to an ascending type mediastinitis, the most reported are: appendectomy, bariatric surgery, as well as gastric perforations secondary to funduplicature, liver abscesses, pyocholecystitis and intestinal perforations with or without diaphragmatic hernia. [5,19,24].

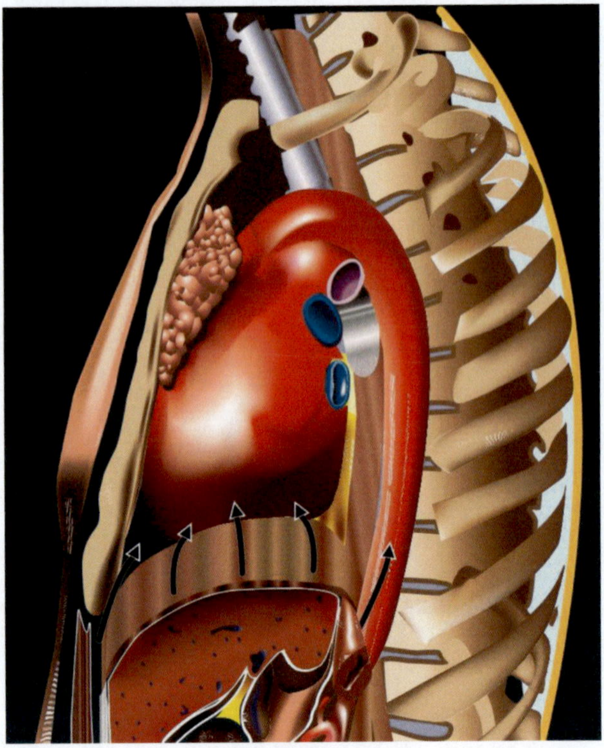

Figure 3. Schematic representation of the thorax demonstrating the pathways of peritoneal and retroperitoneal septic processes through their fascia and anatomic relationship (arrows).

Diagnosis

Diagnosis is performed through a complete medical history and physical examination. If there is a suspected torpid evolution of the abdominal infectious process, a simple chest x-ray is warranted. A thoraco-abdominal contrast enhanced CT must be also performed (Figure 4), with follow up in the intensive care unit with close follow-up in case this complication arises, and it could be addressed in a timely manner avoiding, to every extent, a septic shock that would lead to multiple organ failure and death. [2,4,5, 9,12,15,18]

Once ascending mediastinitis criteria are met by radiologic imaging and laboratory studies establishing a diagnosis of sepsis and an acute systemic inflammatory response with a cephalic infectious spread, it is of the outmost importance that the thoracic surgery team be involved in the treatment protocol to immediately refer the patient to the OR. [1,3,12,14]

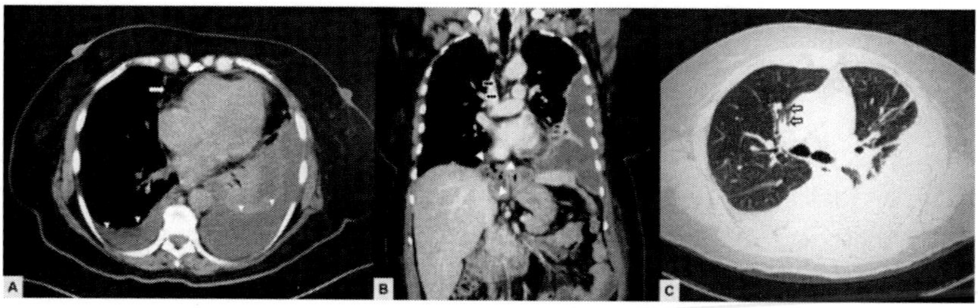

Figure 4. (A) Axial tomographic view demonstrating retrosternal gas (*arrow*) and bilateral pleural effusions (*arrowheads*). (B) Coronal tomographic reconstruction demonstrating a left pleural effusion with passive atelectasis and gas at the periphery of the superior vena cava (*arrows*), and purulent effusion with gas in the esophageal hiatus (*arrowheads*). (C) Axial pulmonary window where gas can be seen in the vicinity of the superior vena cava (arrows) in a patient that previously was treated for an emphysematous pyelonephritis. (Reproduced with permission).

Treatment

The surgical approach must be a multidisciplinary process, being mandatory, control of thoracic and abdominal infections, with aggressive and early treatment for sepsis control. To achieve this, an open abdominal wound could be an option, with the use of negative pressure wound therapy (NPWT). [2]

Simultaneously, thoracic drainage is advised. We recommend performing it through a right thoracotomy with drainage and debridement of the mediastinum having an exhaustive surgical lavage by communicating both pleural spaces and leaving the operated chest with 2 right and a left single pleural tubes as described in previous chapters; there is also a documented case of drainage through thoracoscopy with a successful outcome. Since these are complex cases, intensive therapy management should focus on wide spread antibiotics treating for anaerobic gram-positive and gram-negative bacteria, adequate electrolyte management, strict control of septic shock and control of the inflammatory response. It is important to take into account the respiratory complications which are the most frequent causes of morbidity and mortality. It is imperative that clinicians have proper coordination with the thoracic and abdominal surgical teams since the patient may require several interventions. [3,5-7,9,10,12,14,15,17,18,20,22-26]

Conclusion

Ascending necrotizing mediastinitis is a diagnostic and therapeutic challenge that needs a multidisciplinary approach specialized on the management of a septic process and control of the inflammatory systemic response, it demands complete mediastinal drainage with debridement via a thoracotomy or a video-assisted thoracoscopic surgery (VATS). These patients need to be controlled in the Intensive Care Unit; the severity index scores that the authors have used to predict for morbidity and mortality are APACHE-IV and SAPS-3 scores, however they have not proven their accuracy yet, as for now it is safe to say that they are reliable for having a general picture of the patient´s metabolic state regarding the infectious process. The most important method to observe and follow-up the septic process in these patients, is through a contrast-enhanced CT; although, it is important to note that up until this day, mortality keeps high even with all the technological advances of the past years.

References

[1] Deu-Martin M, Saez-Barba M, López-Sanz I, Alcaraz-Peñarrocha R, Romero-Vielva L, Solé-Montserrat J. Factores de riesgo de mortalidad

en la mediastinitis necrosante descendente. *Arch Bronconeumol* 2010;46:182-187.

[2] Horan TC1, Andrus M, Dudeck MA. CDC/NHSN surveillance definition of health care-associated infection and criteria for specific types of infections in the acute care setting. *Am J Infect Control* 2008;36(5):309-332.

[3] Dajer-Fadel WL, Pichardo-González M, Estrada-Ramos S, Palafox D, Navarro-Reynoso FP, Argüero-Sánchez R. Ascending necrotizing mediastinitis secondary to emphysematous pyelonephritis. *Asian Cardiovasc Thorac Ann* 2014;22(7):869-871.

[4] Edwin F1, Tettey MM, Tamatey M, Frimpong-Boateng K. eComment: Optimal exposure for debridement of necrotizing mediastinitis and bilateral empyema thoracis. *Interact Cardiovasc Thorac Surg* 2009;9(1):146.

[5] Zacate-Otero T, Montiel-Jarquin A, Salazar-Ibarguen J, López-Colombo A. Complicaciones de la cirugía antirreflujo. *Cir Ciruj* 2001;69(2):57-61.

[6] Khaleghnejad-Tabari A, Mirshemirani A, Rouzrokh M, Mohajerzadeh L, Khaleghnejad-Tabari N, Ghaffari P. *Acute Mediastinitis in Children: A Nine-Year Experience Tanaffos* 2013;12(2):48-52.

[7] Nullmeier S, Kuhn R, Lippert H, Motsch C. Ascending pancreatitis with mediastinal and parapharyngeal involvement. *HNO* 2009;57(9):965-968.

[8] Ahmed-Nusrath A, Nusrath MA, Annamaneni R. Faecal mediastinitis following decompression of suspected tension pneumothorax. *Emerg Med J* 2007; 24(12): 830.

[9] Abakumovl MM, Pogodina AN, Barmina TG, Snigirev MV. 20-year experience with diagnosis and treatment of different forms of purulent mediastinitis. *Vestn Khir Im I I Grek* 2001;160(1):80-85.

[10] Holzer R, Pesendorfer FX, Pridun N. Mediastinitis and bilateral pleural effusion of pancreatic origin. *Wien Klin Wochenschr* 1982;94:28–32.

[11] Soto D, Pérez L, González R, Valle V. Mediastinitis secondary to a Zenker diverticulectomy by CO 2 laser. *Rev Esp Anestesiol Reanim* 2013;60(7):418.

[12] Marty-Ané CH, Berthet JP, Alric P, Pegis JD, Rouvière P, Mary H. Management of descending necrotizing mediastinitis: an aggressive treatment for an aggressive disease. *Ann Thorac Surg* 1999;68:212-217.

[13] Hasegawa T, Endo S, Sohara Y. Classification of descending necrotizing mediastinitis. *Ann Thorac Surg* 2000;69:1295–1302.

[14] Ronson RS, Duarte I, Miller JI. Embryology and surgical anatomy of the mediastinum with clinical implications. *Surg Clin North Am* 2000;80(1):157-169.

[15] Chang YC, Chen CW. Thoracoscopic drainage of ascending mediastinitis arising from pancreatic pseudocyst. *Interact Cardiovasc Thorac Surg* 2009;9:144–146.

[16] Corsten MJ, Shamji FM, Odell PF, Frederico JA, Laframboise GG, Reid KR, Vallieres E, Matzinger F. Optimal treatment of descending necrotising mediastinitis. *Thorax* 1997;52:702–708.

[17] Hasegawa T, Endo S, Sohara Y. Classification of descending necrotizing mediastinitis. *Ann Thorac Surg* 2000;69:1295–1302.

[18] Dajer-Fadel WL, Ramírez-Castañeda S, Flores-García M, Flores-Calderón O, Mejía-Melgar EM, Tortolero-Sánchez CR, Argüero-Sánchez R, Ibarra-Pérez C. Pericarditis purulenta, un caso exitoso. *Rev Med Hosp Gen Mex* 2013;76(4):195-199.

[19] Chávez EJI, González MMA, González SR, Cortés GE, Sánchez CRM, Chávez FA. Patología pleural, modalidad clínico-quirúrgica. *Rev Hosp Jua Mex* 2005;72(4):139-147.

[20] Cho JS, Kim YD, Hoseok I, Lee SK, Jeong YJ. Treatment of mediastinitis using video-asisted thoracoscopic surgery. *Eur J Cardiothorac Surg* 2008;34:520–524.

[21] Dajer-Fadel WL, Ibarra-Pérez C, Sánchez-Velazquez LD, Borrego-Borrego R, Navarro-Reynoso FP, Argüero-Sánchez R. Descending necrotizing mediastinitis below the tracheal carina. *Asian Cardiovasc Thorac Ann* 2014;22(2):176-182.

[22] Ayuso-Velasco R, García-Barajas S, García-Sáez M. Mediastinitis secondary to acute pancreatitis. *Arch Bronconeumol* 2011;47(6):319-320.

[23] Iacono C1, Procacci C, Frigo F, Andreis IA, Cesaro G, Caia S, Bassi C, Pederzoli P, Serio G, Dagradi A. Thoracic complications of pancreatitis. *Pancreas* 1989;4(2):228–236.

[24] Mejía-Melgar EM, Dajer-Fadel WL, Tortolero-Sánchez CR, Ramírez-Montaño L, Borrego-Borregoc R, Navarro-Reynoso FP, Ibarra-Pérez C, Argüero-Sánchez R. Tratamiento exitoso de un caso de perforación esofágica posterior. *Rev Med Hosp Gen Mex* 2014;77(1):37-42.

[25] Macrí P1, Jiménez MF, Novoa N, Varela G. A descriptive analysis of a series of patients diagnosed with acute mediastinitis. *Arch Bronconeumol* 2003;39(9):428-430.

[26] Dajer-Fadel WL, Ibarra-Pérez C, Argüero-Sánchez R. Mediastinal drainage in descending necrotizing mediastinitis. *Asian Cardiovasc Thorac Ann* 2013;21:493-495.

In: Mediastinal Infections
Editor: Walid Leonardo Dajer-Fadel
ISBN: 978-1-63463-369-7

Chapter 8

Post-Operative Mediastintis

R. Argüero-Sánchez[1*], A. Ramírez-Castañeda[2], S. Ramírez-Castañeda[1] and W. L. Dajer-Fadel[1]
[1]Cardiothoracic Surgery Department,
General Hospital of Mexico
"Dr. Eduardo Liceaga", Mexico City, Mexico
[2]Cardiology Hospital of the National Medical Center "Siglo XXI",
IMSS, Mexico City, Mexico

Abstract

Post-operative mediastinitis is one of the most feared complications when performing a cardiac surgery through a sternotomy, compared to other types of surgery, this one exposes the most the cardiac tissue to the thoracic surface, with increased risk for infection in diabetic, obese or patients with chronic renal insufficiency, among others; as any post-operative infection, the causative agents are usually from normal skin flora such as *Staphylococcus aureus* and *Staphylococcus epidermidis*, therefore, preventive measures before, during and after surgery are discussed in extent to achieve adequate results and decrease the possibilities of allowing microbial growth within the incision, sometimes limited to superficial planes, but in other instances these can advance to more deep layers.

* Correspondence to: Rubén Argüero-Sánchez, E-mail address: rubenarguero@gmail.com.

In the second part of this chapter, diagnosis and treatment are analyzed, emphasizing how in recent years the use of negative pressure wound therapy has revolutionized prognosis in these patients, reducing mortality as low as 4%, also older techniques are reviewed since they are still valid for a mixed management of deep sternal infections. It is important to take every angle into consideration when dealing with patients with post-operative mediastinitis (PM) since every detail is important, and catastrophic outcomes are seen when overlooking them, the sooner the identification of the infection, the faster the patient will receive appropriate care improving its prognosis.

Etiology

Deep sternal infections are present in approximately 1.2% of patients after a cardiac procedure. [1] Despite the use of sterile techniques, preoperative antibiotics and adequate wound care. Infections originated at the sternal wound evolve to mediastinitis in 1-3% of the cases. [2] PM, also called deep infection of the sternum, is one of the most feared complications in heart surgery.

Although, incidence being low, there is a high mortality associated with it that spans from 10 to 25%. [3] This infection is more seen in male patients about 70% of the time and age >60 years-old. [3, 4]

The most commonly associated microorganisms are *Staphylococcus epidermidis* and *Staphylococcus aureus*, both being a part of normal skin flora, they are involved in 43-64% of the cases, as seen in recent studies; however no difference in mortality was found when caused by one pathogen or another compared to other microorganisms such as gram-negative bacteria. [5] *S. aureus* is reported to develop a more aggressive form of disease and is also associated with the most classical signs of mediastinal infection. This microorganism is identified with the colonization of nasal airways; the incidence is about 10-15% which is associated with an increased risk of PM. [6]

Another study identified these bacteria to be in 75% out of the 79% gram-positive cultured bacteria, whilst gram-negative bacteria where 19% out of 146 cases. [4]

Individual Studies (Tables 1, 2 & 3) Where Diferent Microoganisms Were Identified

Table 1. Microorganisms cultured in post-operative mediastinitis out of 146 patients. [4]

Bacteria	Patient n	Percentage
Staphylococcus aureus	46	31.5
Staphylococcus epidermidis	65	44.5
Streptococcus viridans	3	2
Enterococcus	2	1.4
Enterobacter cloacae	12	8.2
Serratia marcescens	6	4.1
Morganella Morgagni	3	2
Proteus mirabilis	3	2
Klebsiella pneumonia	3	2
Other unknown microorganisms	2	1.3

Table 2. Microorganisms cultured in post-operative mediastinitis in 132 patients [2]

Bacteria	Patient n	Percentage
Staphylococcus aureus	72	55
Negative-coagulase Staphylococcus	19	14
Pseudomonas aeruginosa	4	3
Enterococcus faecalis	4	3
Proteus mirabilis	3	2
Serratia marcescens	3	2
Escherichia coli	3	2
Enterococcus faecium	2	2
Klebsiella pneumonia	1	1
Methicillin resistant Staphylococcus aureus	1	1
Enterococcus casselliflavus	1	1
Enterobacter cloacae	1	1
Mycoplasma hominis	1	1
Bacteroides capillosus	1	1
Morganella morganii	1	1
Corynebacterium	1	1
Enterobacter aerogenes	1	1

In some cases infections could present with more than one pathogen. The mean time of antibiotic treatment was 33.1 ± 15.3 days. [7] When a superficial wound dehiscence is evident after a heart surgery it is considered a minor complication, it is relatively frequent and requires prolonged medical care. Debridement with wound closure are valid and safe procedures for the treatment of these patients. [8]

Table 3. Microorganisms cultured in post-operative mediastinitis in 124 patients [7]

Bacteria from mediastinal process	Percentage
Staphylococcus aureus	51.6
Coagulase-negative Staphylococcus	22.6
Enterococos faecalis	6.5
Pseudomonas aeruginosa	5.6
Serratia marcescens	3.2
Proteus mirabilis	2.4
Enterococcus faecium	2.4
Enterobacter aerogenes, Morganella morganii, E. Coli	Few patients
No growth in cultures (previous antibiotic treatment)	3.2

Table 4. Incidence of post-operative mediastinitis according to performed surgery in 132 patients. [2]

Procedure	Percentage
Previous surgery	26 - 49
Coronary artery bypass grafting	72 - 85
Left internal thoracic artery harvested	67 - 83
Right internal thoracic artery harvested	10 - 28
Aortic valve replacement	19 - 29
Mitral valve replacement or repair	7 - 9
Surgical time (minutes)	173±71 - 246±76
Cardiovascular bypass time (minutes)	99±50 - 128±74
Aortic cross-clamp time (minutes)	65±38 - 86±61

Procedures Associated to Mediastinitis

As inferred from previous paragraphs PM is usually associated to revascularization surgery, however this is not true in every case, in table four we present an analysis of mayor causes for this disease, it is important for the thoracic surgeon to be aware of these since most of the time medical decisions are based on how frequent PM is associated with a certain procedure, and as specialists on the subject there should be a very short margin of error. [2]

It has been continuously emphasized that the use of mammary arteries during cardiac surgery is a clear risk factor for this disease; however it could be acceptable to proceed when deciding whether or not this intervention is beneficial for the patient despite the threat.

Risk Factors

The factors associated to PM are: duration of surgery, use of both internal thoracic arteries, excessive transfusion of blood products, prolonged mechanical ventilation, pulmonary or gastrointestinal complications. [4,9] Case-control studies have shown that obese patients, tobacco use, chronic obstructive pulmonary disease, diabetes mellitus, peripheral vascular disease and congestive cardiac insufficiency are at increased risk for PM. Also those with a reduced left ventricle ejection fraction, coronary bypass surgery patients, use of internal thoracic artery, need for an intra-aortic balloon pump, or re-operations for ischemia / bleeding. In another study, no difference was found as risk factor for PM regarding aortic cross-clamp or perfusion time. The incidence for PM in patients operated for revascularization alone, cardiac valve surgery alone, or combined was 2.8% (106/3737), 1.1% (14/1334), and 3.2% (25/811) respectively. [4] There is no clear evidence of the pathophysiology involved in obese patients (BMI > 30 kg/m^2), however, it is hypothesized that perioperative antibiotics could have a sub-optimal distribution in adipose tissue, also the depth of this layer obscures diagnosis of PM, when in thin patients it is quickly evident in the post-operative period. [10]

Inaccurate antiseptic measures could play a role in the pathologic mechanism of infection, more so in patients that need to undergo a redo-surgery due to life-threatening hemorrhage, and in some cases these measures are overlooked due to the urgency of the procedure. [11,12] High levels of blood glucose have also demonstrated bad wound healing, this was demonstrated when strict control was implemented with insulin in diabetic patients, the incidence of PM decreased. [13]

A low left ventricle ejection fraction (<30%) and congestive cardiac insufficiency with a high functional class value of the New York Heart

Association are also risk factors for PM. [14] A low ejection fraction alone has also been proposed as an independent risk factor by various associations and included in the most recent guidelines. [15] The use of bone wax during cardiac surgery has been proved that is not an independent risk factor for PM despite many doubts and controversies of the past. [16]

Using univariate analysis, as expected, 90-day-mortality was higher for patients with PM (14.5%) compared to non-PM patients (2.8%), reporting an early death risk for mortality in those with renal chronic insufficiency and previous heart surgery. There are other factors that influence mortality related to the procedure, such as increased Intensive Care Unit length of stay, postoperative renal insufficiency and the need for blood components transfusion. The variables related infection with early mortality was the use of wound tissue interposition during the first reoperation, presence of concomitant bacteria, and presence of *S. aureus* in culture results. [4]

Prevention of Post-Operative Mediastinitis According to Risk Factors

Minimizing risk factors for every procedure is very important. A strict control in diabetics during or after surgery is always warranted, preoperative glucose should be controlled with hemoglobin A_1C levels. Also antiplatelet drugs such as aspirin and clopidogrel are to be taken into account; although results have been controversial and complex. [18-22] We will now discuss the related literature to other preventable preoperative risk factors that have been the subject of debate over the years.

Preoperative screening for nasal S. aureus and the use of mupirocin nasal ointment: Many issues have risen in the past regarding this practice, the main ones are drug efficacy, follow-up on culture results, potential for a widespread high-level resistance to mupirocin, and cost. On the other hand, the rationale for preoperative screening and treatment with mupirocin are: a) 40 – 80% of wound infections are due to *S.aureus* with increasing number of patients with methicillin resistant *Staphylococcus aureus* (MRSA) which carry a higher risk of morbidity and death; these patients have a tendency of being older and have more comorbidities. [23,24] b) Infections usually arise from the patients´ own flora, with enough evidence suggesting colonization with this microbe preceding deep wound infections, [25] and finally c) there is abundant data that patients treated with 2% mupirocin before surgery decrease surgical wound infections. [26] Two modes of action have been adopted in cardiac surgery centers which are: "treat-all" or "screen-all" patients for MRSA; according to Bryan *et al.* [27] it makes sense to implement this practice in hospitals that have known past evidence of high incidence with infections cultured by this bacteria. This policy is considered logical since there is sufficient data suggesting that a rise in drug resistance can be seen when treating patients with mupirocin. [28] Another issue is costs and logistic of management, since patients need to be treated five days before the surgery; cost-effectiveness studies have shown that this practice augments the number of medical visits and laboratory use for diagnosis. [29]

Preoperative bathing: A known fact is that bathing before surgery reduces bacterial colonization, however three randomized controlled trials and a meta-analysis have not been able to reject the null hypothesis regarding wound infection rate in the postoperative period, [30] therefore this is no longer an accepted practice for the prevention of PM.

Prophylactic antibiotic therapy: the benefits of this practice have been proved many times, current guidelines suggest that a cephalosporin, usually cefazolin or cefuroxime should be given within 60 minutes before the skin incision and continued for no longer than 48 hours. [31] An alternative drug for allergic patients when β-lactam agents or MRSA are suspected, is the use of vancomycin.

Reducing Risk Factors during Surgery

Many risk factors have been historically considered during cardiac surgery, the most important ones will be discussed, for instance a sterile operating room should be always sought, with an adequate ventilation system to avoid *Aspergillus* and *Legionella* infections; a well-trained team in hygienic operating-room practices and adherence to basic surgical principles, like control of bleeding (due to the propensity of infection when this is excessive), accurate anatomic dissection, the use of completely sterile equipment, good operative techniques, exact approximation of wound tissues without excessive tightness, and gentle tissue handling.

Internal thoracic arteries: Risk of infection due to poor wound site vascular irrigation has been controversial and the only study that reduced this incidence showed that the use of rigid-plates for sternal fixation accomplishes its purpose. [32]

Glycemic control: When hyperglycemia is present many things happen; pathogen proliferation and impaired neutrophil function, among others; some authors find these statements controversial, nevertheless many others affirm that an intraoperative hyperglycemic state with an increased serum glucose in a mean of 20 mg/dL correlates with a 30% probability for complications (infection among them), this findings where confirmed by other groups as well, with a higher death, length of stay and infection rates; and that the risk was eliminated by reducing glucose with continuous insulin infusion. [33-35]

Other practices of prevention: Among many clinical trials that try to reduce risk of infection during cardiac surgery, just a few succeeded. Yoshii *et al.* prospered in this task by spraying antibiotic solution containing cefazolin and gentamicin into the operative field.

Vander Salm *et al.* applied topical vancomycin to the sternal edges reducing infection rates. Other groups have used a gentamicin-collagen sponge, leaving it in the sternal wound reducing infection rates from 3.6% to 0.6%, however these results where contradicted by two systematic reviews. Maclver *et al.* applied bacitracin to the sternotomy with apparent effective results. Many of these practices seem promising, however they still need external validation studies and randomized controlled trials to prove their effectiveness, but surely clinical investigation addressing this issue should never stop until thriving for better results each time. [36-40]

Reducing Postoperative Risk Factors

Logically proper hygienic maintenance of the Intensive Care Unit and Cardiovascular Recovery Room are essential because previous patients with infectious processes increase the risk of new infections for incoming patients.

Desirable evidence based practices included in this important stage of care is: early extubation, early central venous and peripheral catheter withdrawal, insulin infusion in diabetics, daily clinical wound evaluation for early infection detection and early reoperation for bleeding. Regarding the use of other antibiotics apart from the recommended have not demonstrated a reduction in complications. [41-47].

It is the authors´ practice and a suggestion to the reader, reduction of global risks for infection in PM should continuously be assessed by the members of the team involving personnel from in the Outpatient Clinic, ICU, anesthesiologists, perfusionists, nurses and physicians rather than only the surgeons; continuously advocating that a new hospital policy should be implemented (based on evidence) when necessary and feasible.

Diagnosis and Classification

Superficial infections after cardiac surgery are defined as an invasion of the subcutaneous and soft tissues without extension to the periosteum. For a deep infection to be diagnosed, it should present at least one of the following: [17]

a) Identification of a pathogenic organism in culture or mediastinal fluid.
b) Evidence of mediastinitis during surgical exploration.
c) One of the following conditions: thoracic pain, sternal instability, fever above 38.8°C, in combination with mediastinal purulent exudate, positive blood cultures or mediastinal fluid drainage for a microorganism.

Sometimes infection is very evident during exploration (Figure 1), but in order to plan a treatment and further study this disease, it is necessary to classify PM; in table 4 this is shown. [4,48]

The severity of PM is categorized according to the level of involved tissues, these are: 1) subcutaneous tissue, 2) sternum, and 3) pericardial sac (table 5). [2]

Table 5. Post-operative mediastinitis classification

Type	Characteristics
I	During the first two weeks after surgery, without risk factors
II	Between weeks 2 - 6 after surgery in absence of risk factors
III a	Type I with the presence of one or more risk factors
III b	Type II with the presence of one or more risk factors
IV a	Type I, II or III after one failed treatment for mediastinitis
IV b	Type I, II or III after more than one failed treatment for mediastinitis
V	When disease is evident for the first time after post-operative week 6

The common signs of sternal infection are fever, leukocytosis, persistence of purulent exudate, pain and sternal instability. [49] It is essential to warn the patients about exudate from the wound, sternal dehiscence or chest instability;

if this occurs in the upper third of the sternum is most worrisome compared to lower portions of the anterior thorax. When these signs are present, they should receive attention without wasting time.

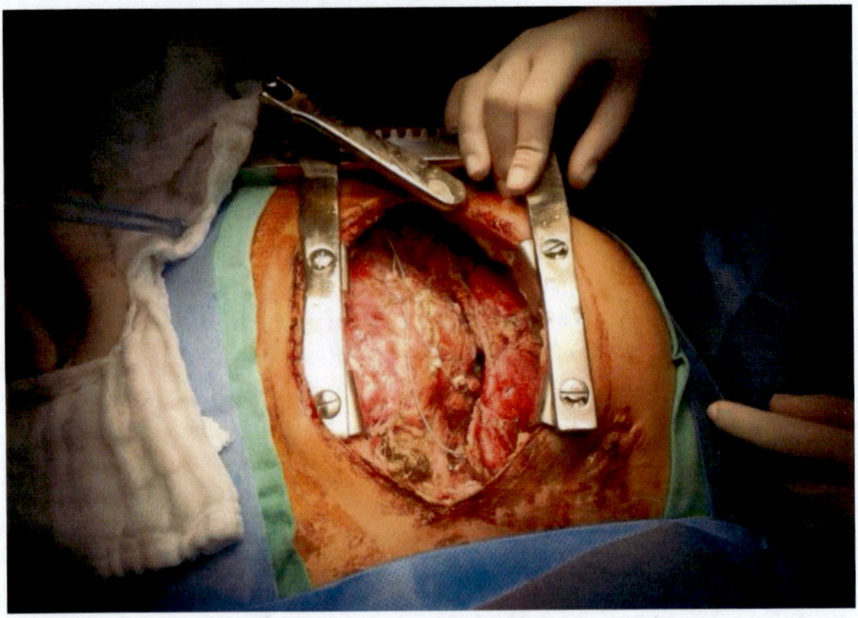

Figure 1. Cephalic trans-operative view during exploration of a post-operative mediastinitis, an active infectious process can be seen in the anterior mediastinum with fibrotic and necrotic tissue among the fascia.

In further chapters we will discuss the tomographic correlation with these complications which is the standard of care for diagnosis; also C-reactive protein is useful to evaluate these cases. [50]

Prognosis

MP incidence is considered relatively low, it spans between 1-3%, however, mortality is considerably high (10-35%). [3, 12] In recent years short-term results have improved, however, in the long-term they are significantly different. [4] When PM has reached deep layers mortality can reach up to 70%; on the brighter side, recent literature on the subject has conveyed better results. [51] Hospital length of stay is severely affected in these patients. [3]

Many treatment modalities have been reported and will be discussed in the following chapters, but it is important to highlight how standard of care has been modified from the past until recent times, gradually improving outcomes as time passes; initially treated by an exploratory sternotomy and packing the cavity with gauzes, exchanging them in the following days with an open wound; once improvement is evident, the next step would be to reconstitute thoracic structural anatomy by means of wires or leaving the wound opened for second intention closure; unfortunately with this technique mortality was reported to be as high as 45%. [52]

The latest reports on the use of negative pressure wound therapy (NPWT) have demonstrated a marked improvement in mortality compared with older techniques (debridement of necrotized tissue, sternal wires removal, irrigation and lavage of the mediastinum, omental transposition or sternal re-suturing), reducing it from 41.7% to 12.4%; [53] In some studies this has been reduced to 4.8%. [1] Also the use of Redon drainage has a reported mortality of 8.9% in PM. [8] When this infection is present not only mortality is high, but also morbidity. [54]

Also, the use of NPWT has been employed as bridge to placement of a tissue flap on the wound once its without infection, this technique reported a 3.7% mortality rate; [55] this is why the use of this technology for preserving the sternum followed by late closure and the use of muscular or omental flaps, have been proposed as the standard of care. [1]

Conclusion

As we learned from the chapter, prevention and applying the necessary steps to avoid mediastinal infections are important points for achieving a seamless progression in operated patients.

There are several microorganisms responsible for this type of mediastinitis, inarguably *S. aureus* and *S. epidermidis* are the most common ones; once diagnosis is made according current guidelines, the use of NPWT has demonstrated to be the standard of care, alone or in conjunction with other techniques such as muscle transposition or omental flap placement after a confirmed clean wound.

When differentiating this disease with other types of mediastinitis, new technology has truly helped these patients with NPWT achieving a reported mortality as low as 4%, an encouraging result when compared to other infections of the mediastinum that have not been modified in the last 50 years. In figure 2 we suggest a treatment algorithm for these cases.

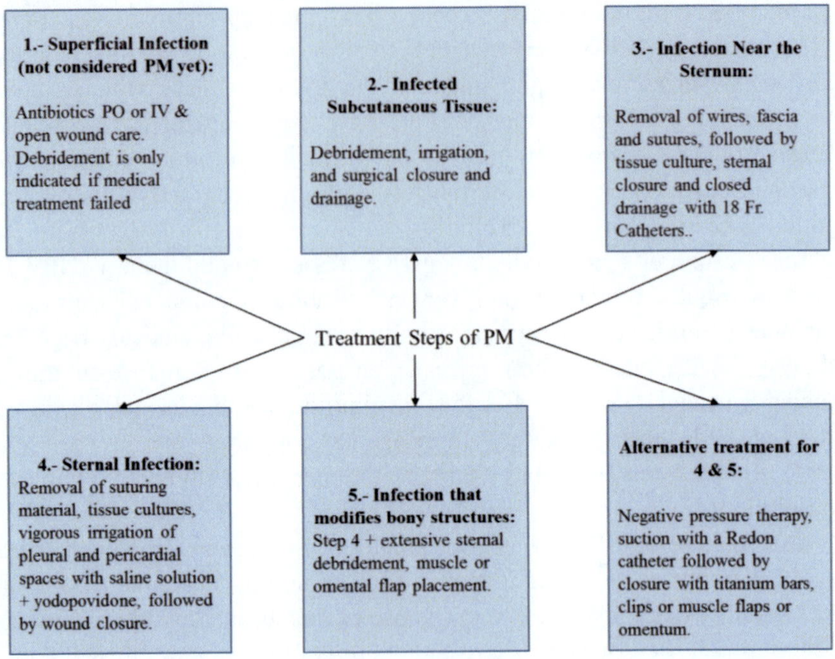

Figure 2. Suggested algorithm for the treatment of post-operative mediastinitis ordered by steps according to severity of the infection.

References

[1] Baillot I, Cloutier D, Montalin L, Co^te´ L, Lellouche F, Houde Ch, Gaudreau G, Voisine P. A total of 161 patients developed mediastinitis (0.84%) Impact of deep sternal wound infection management with vacuum-assisted closure therapy followed by sternal osteosynthesis: a 15-year review of. *Eur J of Cardiothorac Surg* 2010;37:880-887.

[2] Roemer J. Vosa, Yilmaza A, Sonkera U, Johannes C. Kelderb, Kloppenburga G. Primary closure using Redon drains vs vacuum-assisted closure in post-sternotomy mediastinitis *Eur J Cardiothorac Surg* 2012;42:e53–e57.

[3] Sjogren J, Malmsjo M, Gustafsson R, Ingemansson R. Poststernotomy mediastinitis: a review of conventional surgical treatments,vacuum-assisted closure therapy and presentation of the Lund University Hospital mediastinitis algorithm. *Eur J of Cardiothorac Surg* 2006;30:898-905.
[4] Poncelet A, Lengele B, Delaere B, Zech F, Glineur D, Funken J, El Khoury G, Noirhomme Ph. Algorithm for primary closure in sternal wound infection: a single institution 10-year experience. *Eur J Cardiothoracic Surg* 2008;33:232-238.
[5] Gardlund B, Bitkover CY, Vaage J. Postoperative mediastinitis in cardiacsurgery—microbiology and pathogenesis. *Eur J Cardiothorac Surg* 2002;21:825-830.
[6] Jakob HG, Borneff-Lipp M, Bach A, von PS, Windeler J, Sonntag H, Hagl S. The endogenous pathway is a major route for deep sternal wound infection. *Eur J Cardiothorac Surg* 2000;17:154-160.
[7] Vosa R, van Putteb B, Sonkera U, and Geoffrey T.L. Kloppenburga. Primary closure using Redon drains for the treatment of post-sternotomy mediastinitis. *Interactive CardioVasc and Thorac Surg* 2014;18:33–37.
[8] Zeitani J, MD, Bertoldo F, MD, Bassano C, MD, PhD, Penta de Peppo A, MD, Pellegrino A, MD, Fadi M. El Fakhri, MD, and Chiariello L, MD. Superficial Wound Dehiscence After Median Sternotomy: Surgical Treatment Versus Secondary Wound Healing. *Ann Thorac Surg* 2004;77:672–675.
[9] Toumpoulis IK, Anagnostopoulos CE, DeRose Jr. JJ, Swistel DG. The impact of deep sternal wound infection on long-term survival after coronary artery bypass grafting. *Chest* 2005;127:464-471.
[10] Milano CA, Kesler K, Archibald N, Sexton DJ, Jones RH. Mediastinitis after coronary artery bypass graft surgery. Risk factors and long-term survival. *Circulation* 1995;92:2245-2251.
[11] Ottino G, De PR, Pansini S, Rocca G, Tallone MV, Comoglio C, Costa P,Orzan F, Morea M. Major sternal wound infection after open-heart surgery: a multivariate analysis of risk factors in 2,579 consecutive operative procedures. *Ann Thorac Surg* 1987;44:173-179.
[12] Lu JC, Grayson AD, Jha P, Srinivasan AK, Fabri BM. Risk factors for sternal wound infection and mid-term survival following coronary artery bypass surgery. *Eur J Cardiothorac Surg* 2003; 23:943-949.
[13] Furnary AP, Zerr KJ, Grunkemeier GL, Starr A. Continuous intravenous insulin infusion reduces the incidence of deep sternal wound infection in

diabetic patients after cardiac surgical procedures. *Ann Thorac Surg* 1999; 67:352-360.

[14] Ridderstolpe L, Gill H, Granfeldt H, Ahlfeldt H, Rutberg H. Superficial and deep sternal wound complications: incidence, risk factors and mortality. *Eur J Cardiothorac Surg* 2001;20:1168-1175.

[15] Eagle KA, Guyton RA, Davidoff R, Ewy GA, Fonger J, Gardner TJ, Gott JP, Herrmann HC, Marlow RA, Nugent WC, O'Connor GT, Orszulak TA, RieselbachRE, Winters WL, Yusuf S, Gibbons RJ, Alpert JS, Eagle KA, GarsonJr A, Gregoratos G, Russell RO, Smith Jr. SC. ACC/AHA Guidelines for Coronary Artery Bypass Graft Surgery: A Report of the American College of Cardiology/American Heart Association Task Force on Practice Guidelines (Committee to Revise the 1991 Guidelines for Coronary Artery Bypass Graft Surgery). American College of Cardiology/American Heart Association. *J Am Coll Cardiol* 1999; 34:1262-1347.

[16] Prziborowski J, MD, Hartrumpf M, MD, Stock U, MD, Kuehne R, MD, Albes J, MD, PhD. Is Bone wax Safe and Does It Help? *Ann Thorac Surg* 2008;85:1002–1006.

[17] Crabtree TD, Codd JE, Fraser VJ, Bailey MS, Olsen MA, Damiano Jr RJ.Multivariate analysis of risk factors for deep and superficial sternal infection after coronary artery bypass grafting at a tertiary care medical center *Semin Thorac Cardiovasc Surg* 2004;16:53-61.

[18] Ferraris VA, Ferraris SP, Moliterno DJ, Camp P, Walenga JM, Messmore HL, et al. The Society of Thoracic Surgeons practice guideline series: aspirin and other antiplatelet agents during operative coronary revascularization (executive summary). *Ann Thorac Surg* 2005;79(4):1454–1461.

[19] Ferrandis R, Llau JV, Mugarra A. Perioperative management of antiplatelet-drugs in cardiac surgery. *Curr Cardiol Rev* 2009;5(2):125–132.

[20] Fitchett D, Eikelboom J, Fremes S, Mazer D, Singh S, Bittira B, et al. Dual antiplatelet therapy in patients requiring urgent coronary artery bypass grafting surgery: a position statement of the Canadian Cardiovascular Society. *Can J Cardiol* 2009;25(12):683–689.

[21] Gurbel PA, Mahla E, Tantry US. Peri-operative platelet function testing: the potential for reducing ischaemic and bleeding risks. *Thromb Haemost* 2011;106(2):248–252.

[22] Biancari F, Airaksinen KE, Lip GY. Benefits and risks of using clopidogrel before coronary artery bypass surgery: systematic review

and meta-analysis of randomized trials and observational studies. *J Thorac Cardiovasc Surg* 2012;143(3):665–675.

[23] Combes A, Trouillet JL, Joly-Guillou ML, Chastre J, Gibert C. The impact of methicillin resistance on the outcome of poststernotomy mediastinitis due to Staphylococcus aureus. *Clin Infect Dis* 2004;38(6):822–829.

[24] Reddy SL, Grayson AD, Smith G, Warwick R, Chalmers JA. Methicillin resistant Staphylococcus aureus infections following cardiac surgery: incidence, impact and identifying adverse outcome traits. *Eur J Cardiothorac Surg* 2007;32(1):113–117.

[25] von Eiff C, Becker K, Machka K, Stammer H, Peters G. Nasal carriage as a source of Staphylococcus aureus bacteremia. *N Engl J Med* 2001;344(1):11–16.

[26] Walsh EE, Greene L, Kirshner R. Sustained reduction in methicillin-resistant Staphylococcus aureus wound infections after cardiothoracic surgery. *Arch Intern Med* 2011;171(1): 68–73.

[27] Bryan CS, Yarbrough WM. Preventing deep wound infection after coronary artery bypass grafting. *Tex Heart Inst J* 2013;40(2):125-139.

[28] Cookson BD. The emergence of mupirocin resistance: a challenge to infection control and antibiotic prescribing practice. *J Antimicrob Chemother* 1998;41(1):11–18.

[29] Lee BY, Wiringa AE, Bailey RR, Goyal V, Lewis GJ, Tsui BY, et al. Screening cardiac surgery patients for MRSA: an economic computer model. *Am J Manag Care* 2010;16(7):163–173.

[30] Kamel C, McGahan L, Polisena J, Mierzwinski-Urban M, Embil JM. Preoperative skin antiseptic preparations for preventing surgical site infections: a systematic review. *Infect Control Hosp. Epidemiol* 2012;33(6):608–617.

[31] Engelman R, Shahian D, Shemin R, Guy TS, Bratzler D, Edwards F, et al. The Society of Thoracic Surgeons practice guideline series: antibiotic prophylaxis in cardiac surgery, part II: antibiotic choice. *Ann Thorac Surg* 2007;83(4):1569–1576.

[32] Song DH, Lohman RF, Renucci JD, Jeevanandam V, Raman J. Primary sternal plating in high-risk patients prevents mediastinitis. *Eur J Cardiothorac Surg* 2004;26(2):367–372.

[33] Gandhi GY, Nuttall GA, Abel MD, Mullany CJ, Schaff HV, Williams BA, et al. Intraoperative hyperglycemia and perioperative outcomes in cardiac surgery patients. *Mayo Clin Proc* 2005;80(7):862–866.

[34] Brown JR, Edwards FH, O'Connor GT, Ross CS, Furnary AP. The diabetic disadvantage: historical outcomes measures in diabetic patients undergoing cardiac surgery – the pre-intravenous insulin era. *Semin Thorac Cardiovasc Surg* 2006; 18(4):281–288.

[35] Furnary AP, Wu Y. Eliminating the diabetic disadvantage: the Portland Diabetic Project. *Semin Thorac Cardiovasc Surg* 2006;18(4):302–308.

[36] Yoshii S, Hosaka S, Suzuki S, Takahashi W, Okuwaki H, Osawa H, et al. Prevention of surgical site infection by antibiotic spraying in the operative field during cardiac surgery. *Jpn J Thorac Cardiovasc Surg* 2001;49(5):279–281.

[37] Schimmer C, Ozkur M, Sinha B, Hain J, Gorski A, Hager B, Leyh R. Gentamicin-collagen sponge reduces sternal wound complications after heart surgery: a controlled, prospectively randomized, double-blind study. *J Thorac Cardiovasc Surg* 2012;143(1):194–200.

[38] Creanor S, Barton A, Marchbank A. Effectiveness of a gentamicin impregnated collagen sponge on reducing sternal wound infections following cardiac surgery: a meta-analysis of randomised controlled trials. *Ann R Coll Surg Engl* 2012;94 (4):227–231.

[39] Godbole G, Pai V, Kolvekar S, Wilson AP. Use of gentamicin-collagen sponges in closure of sternal wounds in cardiothoracic surgery to reduce wound infections. *Interact Cardiovasc Thorac Surg* 2012;14(4):390–394.

[40] MacIver RH, Stewart R, Frederiksen JW, Fullerton DA, Horvath KA. Topical application of bacitracin ointment is associated with decreased risk of mediastinitis after median sternotomy. *Heart Surg Forum* 2006;9(5):750–753.

[41] Graf K, Sohr D, Haverich A, Kuhn C, Gastmeier P, Chaberny IF. Decrease of deep sternal surgical site infection rates after cardiac surgery by a comprehensive infection control program. *Interact Cardiovasc Thorac Surg* 2009;9(2):282–286.

[42] Le Guillou V, Tavolacci MP, Baste JM, Hubscher C, Bedoit E, Bessou JP, Litzler PY. Surgical site infection after central venous catheter-related infection in cardiac surgery. Analysis of a cohort of 7557 patients. *J Hosp Infect* 2011;79(3):236–241.

[43] El-Hamamsy I, Durrleman N, Stevens LM, Leung TK, Theoret S, Carrier M, Perrault LP. Incidence and outcome of radial artery infections following cardiac surgery. *Ann Thorac Surg* 2003;76(3):801–804.

[44] Torres S, Kuo YH, Morris K, Neibart R, Holtz JB, Davis JM. Intravenous iron following cardiac surgery does not increase the infection rate. *Surg Infect* (Larchmt) 2006;7(4):361–366.
[45] Elahi MM, Haesey AM, Graham KC, Battula NR, Manketlow B, Dhannapuneni RR, Hickey MS. Leg wound infections following cardiac surgery: a scoring system for assessment and management. *J Wound Care* 2005;14(7):337–340.
[46] Mehta RH, Sheng S, O'Brien SM, Grover FL, Gammie JS, Ferguson TB, et al. Reoperation for bleeding in patients undergoing coronary artery bypass surgery: incidence, risk factors, time trends, and outcomes. *Circ Cardiovasc Qual Outcomes* 2009;2(6):583–590.
[47] Yap EL, Levine A, Strang T, Dunning J. Should additional antibiotics or an iodine washout be given to all patients who suffer an emergency re-sternotomy on the cardiothoracic intensive care unit? *Interact Cardiovasc Thorac Surg*. 2008;7(3): 464–469.
[48] El Oakley RM, Wright JE. Postoperative mediastinitis: classification and management. *Ann Thorac Surg* 1996;61:1030-1036.
[49] Eckstein F, MD, Albes J, MD, Jurmann M, MD, Scheule A, MD, Raygrotzki S, MD, Laniado M, MD, Ziemer G, MD. Surgical Management of Persistent Mediastinitis After Coronary Bypass Grafting. *Ann Thorac Surg* 1997;64:854–856.
[50] Pia Tocco M, Costantino A, Ballardini M, D'Andrea C. Improved results of the vacuum assisted closure and Nitinol clips sternal closure after postoperative deep sternal wound infection. *Eur J Cardiothorac Surg* 2009;35:833-838.
[51] Klesius A, Dzemali O, Simon A, Kleine P, Abdel-Rahman U, Herzog C, Wimmer-Greinecker G, Moritz A. Successful treatment of deep sternal infections following open heart surgery by bilateral pectoralis major flaps. *Eur J Cardiothorac Surgery* 2004;25:218–223.
[52] Sarr MG, Gott VL, Townsend TR. Mediastinal infection after cardiac surgery. *Ann Thorac Surg* 1984;38:415—423.
[53] Grossi EA, Culliford AT, Krieger KH, Kloth D, Press R, Baumann FG, SpencerFC. A survey of 77 major infectious complications of median sternotomy: a review of 7,949 consecutive operative procedures. *Ann Thorac Surg* 1985; 40:214—223.
[54] Vosa R, Yilmaza A, Sonkera U, Kelderb J, Kloppenburga G. Vacuum-assisted closure of post-sternotomy mediastinitis as compared to open packing Interactive. *CardioVascular and Thorac Surg* 2012;14:17–21.

[55] Domkowski PW, Smith ML, Gonyon Jr DL, Drye C, Wooten MK, Levin LS,Wolfe WG. Evaluation of vacuum-assisted closure in the treatment of poststernotomy mediastinitis. *J Thorac Cardiovasc Surg* 2003; 126:386—390.

In: Mediastinal Infections
Editor: Walid Leonardo Dajer-Fadel
ISBN: 978-1-63463-369-7

Chapter 9

Correlative Anatomy in Post-Operative Mediastinitis

O. Flores-Calderón[1*] and S. Ramírez-Castañeda[1,2,3,4,5]

[1] Cardiac Surgery Department, General Hospital of Mexico " Dr. Eduardo Liceaga", Mexico City, Mexico

[2] Cardiology Hospital of the National Medical Center "Siglo XXI", (IMSS), Mexico City, Mexico

[3] General Hospital Adolfo Prieto, Taxco, Guerrero, Mexico

[4] Regional Hospital "Bicentenario de la Independencia" (ISSSTE), Mexico City, Mexico

[5] General Hospital of Acapulco, Guerrero, Mexico

Abstract

Post-operative mediastinitis (PM) is one of the most severe surgical complications with high rates of morbidity and mortality. Their diagnosis are primarily clinical, with systemic inflammatory response, hemodynamic compromise and sepsis. Support diagnostics are done with a computed tomography (CT), however, findings during the first two post-operative weeks may be confused with changes related to the original surgical procedure. Image abnormalities increase according time elapsed after surgery. The main associations found are: a decrease of

* Correspondence to: Octavio Flores-Calderon, E-mail address: caldcronmd@prodigy.net.mx.

mediastinal fat, liquid / air collections, and unilateral or bilateral pleural effusion. The presence of inflammation within the connective and adipose tissues and bilateral pleural effusion suggest mediastinitis. Tomography is more sensitive for detecting sternal dehiscence, sternal erosion or subcutaneous collections. In this chapter we will define radiologic and tomographic findings for the vast majority of patients undergoing cardiac surgery, as well as the main points to determine the correlation in the images for developing infectious processes.

Introduction

Complications related to infectious processes after cardiac surgery occur in 5 to 21% of the cases. When these are severe, mortality increases in more than 5 times extending the time of recovery. In 47% of the cases, these patients require more than 14 days of stay compared a lesser number of days in 5.9% of patients with mild infection. [1]

PM, is one of the most feared surgical complications in cardiothoracic surgery because of its poor prognosis and difficult management, with reported incidences of 0.4% to 5%, with a mortality rate ranging from 7% to 80%, [3,4,5] with a morbidity of up to 50% which leads to an increased hospital length of stay. [2] Diagnostic procedures for PM include physical examination, chest X-ray and cervico-thoracic contrast enhanced CT.

Due to mediastinal anatomical changes and surgical procedure details, post-operative findings can hide an evolving septic process, as well as surgeon´s reluctance to accept the idea that a complication is imminent; so that the diagnosis of PM must be supported not only by radiological but by clinical findings as well.

Post-operative Expected Images

Immediately after cardiac surgery, patients are admitted to the cardiac intensive care unit, and a simple chest X-ray is done. A thorough evaluation of monitor attachments, therapeutic devices, solution balance control, parenchymal abnormalities, cardio-mediastinal silhouette on imaging, liquid collections and extra-pulmonary air are constantly sought. [4]

The cardio-mediastinal silhouette during the post-operative period can be seen slightly larger than preoperatively, in some extent due to the anteroposterior projection taken with a portable X-ray machine, and mainly by the surgical procedure itself (Figure 1). [4] Mediastinal widening in the post-operative period impedes adequate evaluation of complications, since it may disguise edema or bleeding, complicating for diagnosis in mediastinitis. It is also important to note that the presence of air bubbles or liquid collections in the anterior mediastinum could continue present several days or weeks after removal of drains left during surgery. [3]

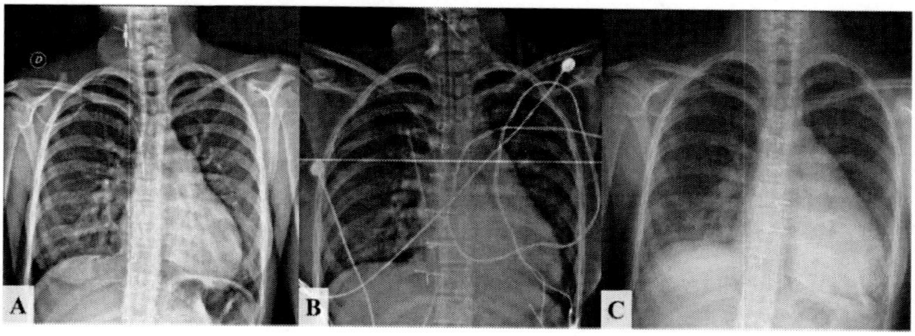

Figure 1. Female patient operated for coronary artery bypass grafting simple chest x-rays before (A), immediately (B) and 16 days after surgery (C) where a widened mediastinum could be seen after the procedure persisting until day 16 as an example of an expected post-operative evolution.

During a sternotomy it is important to preserve the integrity of both mediastinal pleura; however, these could be opened, either incidentally or for drainage purposes when patients have a pleural effusion secondary to their pathological process. This should be considered during the post-operative period, since radiological images of pleural effusion could be seen but considered normal in this type of patients, and not reflecting an infectious state.

Post-operative expected changes in CT can persist for 2-3 weeks which include soft tissue infiltration, edema / blood in the pre-sternal and retro-sternal compartments, and liquid collection as well as a circumscribed hematoma. Air located in the mediastinum is usually reabsorbed up to the 7th day, but may persist for a longer time period. [5-6]

Usually among the post-operative changes, mediastinal adipose tissue is not completely obliterated, some or most of the mediastinal fat radiolucency is preserved. Most patients have an asymmetrical sternum associated with: space between the sternal borders (< 4 mm), bone overlap or impacted bone. Even 6 months after the procedure, only half of the patients have a completely healed sternum, reaching 100% at the end of the first year. [5] Bone callus is not visible by CT until 3 months after surgery. [7]

CT plays a special role in the evaluation of mediastinitis, to estimate the extent and depth of the lesion. The anterior mediastinum is always abnormal after a sternotomy incision. Retro-sternal collections, pneumomediastinum, hematoma, or any combination of these three could be found up until 21 days after surgery in non-complicated patients. [4]

Pathological Findings

When complications arise after a sternotomy they may affect the pre-sternal (cellulitis, abscess), sternal (osteomyelitis, dehiscence) and retrosternal (mediastinitis, hematoma, abscess) compartments. CT plays an important role in evaluating and characterizing post-sternotomy hazards, particularly when assessed two weeks after surgery. [5]

As a result of surgery, mediastinitis is probably the leading cause of the acute type. Sternotomy is the main approach for cardiac surgeries and mediastinal mass removal. [3] According to Reida et al. [2] PM can be divided into 5 types:

1. When it occurs two weeks after surgery, without risk factors.
2. Between post-operative weeks 2 and 6, without risk factors.
3. When it occurs during the first two weeks, with 1 or 2 risk factors.
4. When infection persists after a first course of treatment.
5. When infection occurs for the first 6 weeks after surgery.

Patients with PM may have local signs such as pain, hypersensitivity, erythema and sternal discharge, along with systemic signs such as fever, sepsis, and leukocyte / erythrocyte sedimentation rate increase. [3-5]

The main radiological signs present during PM are: mediastinal widening, gas in the pre-vascular zone, mediastinal air-fluid levels, pneumomediastinum and pleural effusion, which may be related to the surgical procedure performed, however, when it is associated with a poor postoperative evolution, it is mandatory to rule out an incipient mediastinitis. [3]

Patients with a suspected PM should be have a CT done to investigate the presence of mediastinal collections, analyze the density of adjacent soft tissues for edema and determine the extent of the process. In case of spontaneous drainage or exudate through the surgical wound, CT pays an important role in identifying the origin of a superficial *vs.* deep collection, in addition to defining its nature. Collections with <20 Hounsfield Units, indicate a liquid content. However, higher densities are suggestive of blood, without excluding a concomitant infection (Figures 2 and 3). [6]

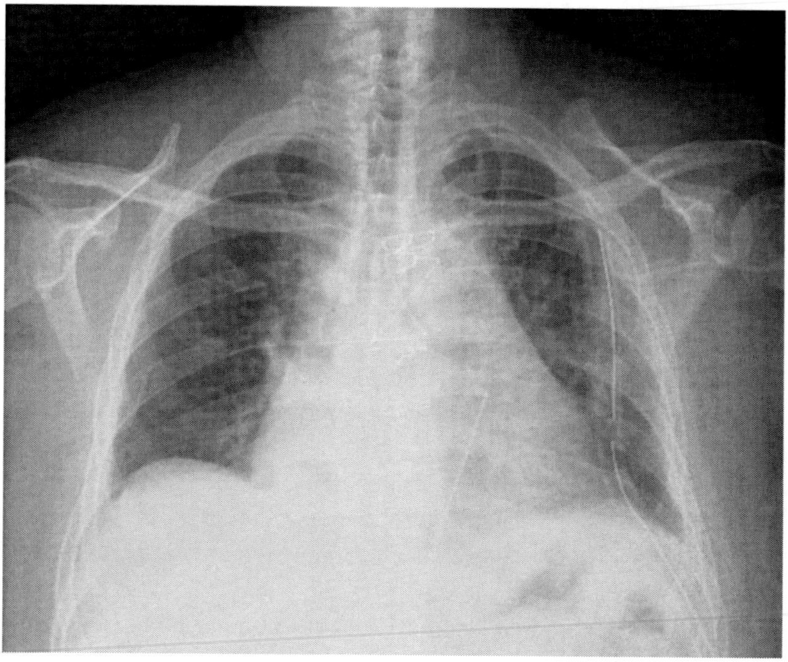

Figure 2. Male patient operated for coronary artery bypass grafting at his first post-operative day with expected changes with a simple x-ray.

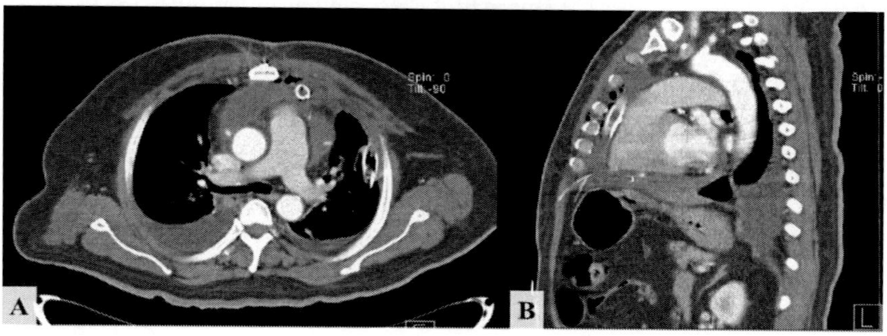

Figure 3. Same patient of figure 2 whom presented fever above 38°C and a deleterious hemodinamic state after 10 days, had a contrast-enhanced computed tomography of the chest performed, noticing in the axial (A) and sagittal (B) views the presence of air bubbles and a para-cardiac collection of 25 HU suggestive of phlegmon.

CT findings can be divided into two large categories: in the mediastinum and on adjacent structures. Mediastinal abnormalities include: collections, air and edema. Regarding adjacent structures: pleural and pericardial effusion, adenopathies, abnormalities of the parenchyma and sternum are also evaluated with this tool. The presence of hypodense collections in the pre- or retro-sternal area in febrile patients is an indication for surgical exploration. [3]

The diagnostic criteria for CT in mediastinitis are the presence of collections in the mediastinum accompanied or not with changes such as edema/densification of soft tissues, sternal separation with bone rim resorption, sclerosis, and sternal osteomyelitis. Other associated findings include lymphadenopathy, cardiac and pleural effusion, subcutaneous emphysema and a consolidated lung. [6] Although, sometimes it is difficult to differentiate tissue changes of inflammation during the early post-operative period, CT helps to evaluate retro-cardiac and sub-phrenic spaces, pleura and superior mediastinum surrounding large vessels. Obviously the presence of air-fluid collections requires exploration and drainage. [8]

The diagnosis of sternal dehiscence may be evident during physical examination. Two major radiological signs are the middle-sternal sign and the displacement of fixation wires; the latter being more accurate. Before it is clinically evident, changes may occur in the distribution of the wires. When a light middle-sternal band is greater than 3 mm, sternal dehiscence should be suspected. [4]

Also, the aid of CT could help to identify complications such as para-median sternotomy and osteomyelitis. The first predisposes to dehiscence, because the thin side of the sternal blade could fracture when closing the wires, with subsequent increase in the space between both sternal tables, evident during this study, [5] this is avoided placing a runing wire in a "zig-zag" fashion between the intercostal spaces parallel to the thin border as a reinforcing "wire rail".

When PM is present after two weeks of surgery, it mainly presents mediastinal collections and sternal alterations such as separation of the blades, marginal bone resorption, sclerosis and signs of partial bone destruction. [6]

Osteomyelitis can be an isolated problem, or it could be associated with dehiscence and subsequent mediastinitis. When found in its early stages, it may be difficult to differentiate from minor sternal irregularities due to osteotomy or other anatomical variants. As it progresses, there will be evident bone destruction, severe demineralization and dehiscence. If diagnosis is still non-conclusive, Gallio-67 could be used as a diagnostic support. [4]

Other signs are mediastinal fat obliteration and diffuse soft tissue infiltration, with or without gas collections. Abscesses easy to diagnose usually are of low density (approximately 20 HU) that may contain gas. Unfortunately, during the immediate post-operative period, when a mediastinitis is in progress, normal edema or air could transpose the images, reducing diagnostic accuracy. However, when these are the findings two weeks post-operatively, they could be highly indicative of mediastinitis. [5] Depending on the depth and extent of the infection, a surgical plan can be done. [9]

Based on what has been said above, the effectiveness of diagnosis is very limited during the first two weeks. [6] A CT scan has a high sensitivity (100%) but low specificity (33%) before the 14th day after surgery. [10] This happens because it is time dependent, making clinical findings essential for diagnosis and management decision. [4, 10] After that period (14 days) CT scans reach 100% sensitivity and specificity. [6] For the medium and long term follow-up, CT is a useful tool to determine the need for antibiotics; also to confirm resolution of the inflammatory process. After surgical drainage, it can identify detritus and areas of possible recurrent infection. [6] In some cases it is also useful as a guide for percutaneous collection drainage. [4]

During the first 10 post-operative days, if a patient develops fever, a retrosternal collection or retro-cardiac abscess may be found. After day 14, a CT helps to evaluate areas of sepsis that were not drained appropriately, demonstrated as collections in the retro-cardiac space or as the presence of empyema. When this happens, signs of mediastinal collections with air may be seen; if the clinical presentation has fewer evident symptoms and signs e.g. drainage of purulent fluid from the mediastinum but with a stable sternum on physical, may be difficult to distinguish from expected changes after surgery. Other areas of interest would be the pleural cavities or the sub-phrenic areas, which merit evaluation by the cardiac surgeon. In all cases a 30 day follow-up is essential to define bone and soft tissue involvement during this process. [8] When an inflammatory mass is seen with a bilateral pleural effussion, it is suggestive of mediastinitis, also when in doubt, a CT helps viewing sternal erosion and subcutaneous collections. [11]

Conclusion

PM is one of the most severe complications after cardiac surgery, with high rates of morbidity and mortality. Anatomical changes related to the surgical procedure hinder the identification of data suggestive of mediastinitis, and may even delay its management in patients that are deemed as inconclusive. The first step in the process of studying a patient begins with evaluation of the clinical evolution with subsequent imaging support with a simple chest X-ray followed by a CT. During the first two weeks, diagnosis is less precise to distinguish between expected post-operative changes from an ongoing mediastinal infection; however, after day 14, sensitivity and specificity increase. Normal CT changes may remain evident until the sixth post-operative month with a logical decrease until they disappear. When suggestive clinical data and CT images are present, the physician should not lose sight of the possibility of dealing with a PM, regardless of the number of days that have passed after surgery. Never forget that imaging studies only serve as a guide only to make the right decision in the appropriate moment.

References

[1] Cove ME, Spelman DW, MacLaren G. Infectious Complications of Cardiac Surgery: A Clinical Review. *J Cardiothorac Vasc Anesth* 2012;22(6):1094-1100.

[2] Careaga-Reyna G, Aguirre-Baca GG, Medina-Concebida LE, Borrayo-Sánchez G, Prado-Villegas G, Argüero-Sánchez R. Risk factors for mediastinitis and sternal dehiscence after cardiac surgery. *Rev Esp Cardiol* 2006;59(2):130-135.

[3] Akman C, Kantarci F, Cetinkaya S. Imaging in mediastinitis: systematic review based on aetiology. *Clinical Radiology* 2004;59:573-585.

[4] Attili I, Kazerooni SA. Postoperative cardiopulmonary thoracic imaging. *Radiol Clin N Am* 2004;42:543-564.

[5] Li AE, Fishman EK. Evaluation of complications after sternotomy using single - and multislice CT with three-dimensional volume rendering. *AJR* 2003;181:1065-1070.

[6] Aguiar de Macedo C, da Silva Baena E, Kato Uezumi K, Campi de Castro C, Luiz Lucarelli C, Guido Cerri G. Acute mediastinitis: multidetector computed tomography findings following cardiac surgery. *Radiol Bras* 2008;41(4):269-273.

[7] Bitkover CY, Cederlund K, Aberg B, Vaage J. Computed tomography of the sternum and mediastinum after median sternotomy. *Ann Thorac Surg* 1999;68:858-863.

[8] Francel TJ, Kouchoukos NT. A rational approach to difficulties after sternotomy wound: the problem. *Ann Thorac Surg* 2001;72:1411-1418.
[9] Bhatnagar G, Vardhanabhuti V, Nensey RR, Sidhu HS, Morgan-Hughes G, Roobottom CA. The role of multidetector computed tomography coronary angiography in imaging complications post-cardiac surgery. *Clinical Radiology* 2013;68:e254-e265.
[10] Nearman H, Klick JC, Eisenberg P, Weighs N. Perioperative complications of cardiac surgery and postoperative care. *Crit Care Clin* 2014;30:527-555.
[11] Misawa Y, Fuse K, Hasegawa T. Infectious mediastinitis after cardiac operations: computed tomographic findings. *Ann Thorac Surg* 1998;65:622-624.

In: Mediastinal Infections
Editor: Walid Leonardo Dajer-Fadel
ISBN: 978-1-63463-369-7

Chapter 10

Surgical Management for Post-Operative Mediastinitis

S. Ramírez-Castañeda*[1,2,3,4*]*, O. Flores-Calderón*[1]*,
***A. Ramírez-Castañeda*[2,5] *and W. L. Dajer-Fadel*[1]**

[1] Cardiac Surgery Department, General Hospital of Mexico " Dr. Eduardo Liceaga", Mexico City, Mexico.
[2] Cardiology Hospital of the National Medical Center "Siglo XXI", (IMSS), Mexico City, Mexico
[3] General Hospital Adolfo Prieto, Taxco, Guerrero, Mexico.
[4] Regional Hospital "Bicentenario de la Independencia" (ISSSTE), Mexico City, Mexico
[5] General Hospital of Acapulco, Guerrero, Mexico

Abstract

Sternotomy wounds due to heart surgery run the risk to get infected in an average of 4%, in spite that patients subject to heart surgery frequently have their thorax opened for several hours causing a major exposure of the wound to the environment, being one of the risk factors for infection development, although appearing only in skin and subcutaneous areas, it is possible to control them with daily wound care and dressing exchange with povidone-iodine; nevertheless, when they appear under a more severe form, i.e., when they are deep, risks are

* Correspondence to: Serafín Ramírez-Castañeda, E-mail address: serafinramir@hotmail.com.

higher due to the close relation of vital structures; therefore, treatment complexity requires early detection, as well as an adequate strategy for the case´s severity. For deep infected post-sternotomy wounds, the arsenal of surgical techniques is ample, such as pectoralis muscles overlapping, although, techniques using the rectus abdominis, external oblique and latissimus dorsi muscles have also been described. As a second line of treatment and an important part of surgical management, are omentoplasty and recently, the use of negative-pressure wound therapy (NPWT).

Introduction

As in other parts of the organism, infections continue to be challenging among patients subjected to heart surgery. Specifically, infected sternotomy incisions and the ones that directly involve the bone, represent an important role for morbidity and mortality.

Infection incidence on soft tissues and sternum ranges from 2.4 - 4% as reported in several series, based on multivariate analysis studies. [1]

There are independent risk factors for infection such as surgery time, cardiopulmonary bypass time, and aortic cross-clamp time, other important factors are the use of internal mammary arteries in patients that are to be revascularized, especially when both vessels are used, with subsequent sternal devascularization [2], reoperation due to bleeding is also an important factor; others are, prolonged intubation due to respiratory complications, diabetes mellitus and massive blood transfusions. [3,4]

In accordance to the guidelines of the Center for Disease Control [5], sternotomy wound infections are classified in superficial when limited to subcutaneous adipose or soft tissues, without involving the periosteum; whereas, deep wound infections that include the sternum require one of the following criteria; an isolated microorganism cultured from mediastinal tissue or fluids, or verifying it during surgery, always accompanied by one of the following data; thoracic pain, sternal instability or fever ≥ 38°C, positive cultures from purulent exudate either through the wound or mediastinal drainages.

Treatment Overview

As for deep wound infections that include the sternum, they have been classified under several forms by Oakley et al. [6] The authors use and treat post-operative mediastinitis using the classification as described by Poncelet Alain et al. [1].

Thus, type I infections are limited to superficial tissues, for which they only require systemic antibiotics and daily wound care with yodopovidone, if this fails, patients shall be taken to the OR so a more complete debridement could be performed, then continued with wound dressings; type II infections also involve subcutaneous layers; systematically, these patients are taken to the OR for debridement and irrigation with yodopovidone, followed by closure and leaving a closed drainage system with suction.

As for type III, they comprise infections next to the bone (sternum), in this scenario, removal of sternal, fascial and subcutaneous sutures with samples taken for culture are warranted, debridement and lavage of all layers are made, followed by closure, leaving an 18 Fr. mediastinal drainage, connected to a closed suction system; as for soft tissues, they are also closed, leaving a 14 Fr drainage system with suction.

When a type IV infection involving the sternal border is present, the same steps mentioned above are performed, a debridement or resection of the sternal border is needed with sampling for cultures, vigorous lavage and drainage of the pleural and pericardial cavities, initially with 4-5 liters of normothermal saline solution, followed by yodopovidone solution, drainages are left in all intervened cavities, and planes are closed in the same manner.

Type V infections include all the previously described characteristics and extensive sternal destruction; for its management, after performing all the steps described above, a wide sternal excision is warranted, where all the affected bone is resected and applying more complex surgical techniques to solve this overwhelming infection, such procedures are described below.

On the next paragraphs the authors offer a description of the techniques for severe degrees in which there is sternal loss, also, as a whole, medical management should include tailored (based on quantitative studies) antibiotic therapy during four to six weeks, as described in the relevant chapter, and with culture controls every week to determine treatment progress, and if necessary, modifying it.

Pectoralis Major Muscle Transposition

This procedure was described and made for the first time in 1976, and ever since it has been positioned as an option for the treatment for deep wounds infected by sternotomy. [7]

The pectoralis muscles transposition as well as plasty with anterior rectus abdominis muscles as a surgical alternative for patients with mediastinitis that have shown failure in previous treatment options that have sustained multiple sternal fractures, as well as with important necrosis and persistence of post-operative mediastinitis. [8, 9]

This procedure may be used as a last surgical alternative even after having used an omental flap lift (omentoplasty) [10] as a primary option or as a reinforcement plasty with major omentum [11, 12], overlapping both sides in the mid-line where they are sutured to provide a force that achieves stability of the thoracic wall [12], besides, the overlapped muscles create a separation between the infected wall and the mediastinum, when associated to an omental flap lifting, they obliterate the dead spaces within the mediastinum, helping prevent fistulas and future wound dehiscence.

Wounds where the top part of the sternum is primarily affected, frequently require only advancement or pectoralis muscle flap in a unilateral or bilateral fashion, in this last case, it is preferred when the mammary arteries are unaffected to avoid necrosis and muscle flap loss. Also when used unilaterally, it is possible to fill the defect entirely, bringing an isolated pectoralis flap, skeletonizing in the proper form the thoraco-acromial vascular pedicle, it is even possible achieving a better advancement by separating and sectioning its humeral insertion [13], although in these cases, it is more probable that complications arise, i,e,. functional problems in shoulder movements such as abduction and internal flexion. [14] Other used techniques of the pectoralis muscle are advancement and rotation, making it the first option when choosing a flap to achieve adequate results in infected sternal wounds, although techniques with rectus abdominis, external oblique and thoracis dorsi muscles have also been described, however left as a second choice, for instance, when both internal thoracic arteries have already been used for coronary grafts (Figure 1). [15]

Experience with overlapping of pectoralis muscles has shown the best results in reference to pain and functional shoulder problems by preserving it; therefore, we will describe the technique for the dissection and overlap of these structures. It is important to mention that in the same way, as in mild infection of soft tissues, where the sternum is preserved, or there is not much tissue destruction or necrosis; devitalized tissue debridement, as well as drainage and thorough lavage with sterile and antiseptic solutions are crucial. Then, infected sternal tissue must be properly resected until finding healthy bone.

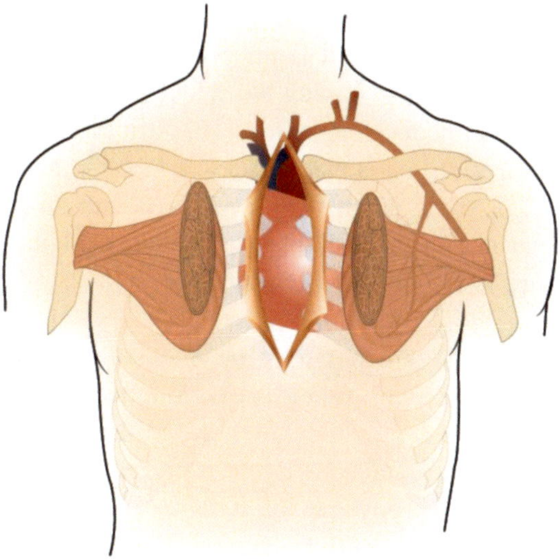

Figure 1. Schematic representation of the pectoralis flaps after dissection for advancement, preserving the thoracoacromial irrigation.

The patient placed in supine position with upper limbs in parallel to the body, should be properly monitored with a central venous line and urinary catheter for better trans-operative control, an available defibrillator should always be in the room, upon inducing anesthesia antiseptic measures are performed, previous sternotomy sutures are removed including wires, the wound is opened with an automatic retractor, proceeding to remove devitalized tissue with scissors and scalpel, cutting until finding viable tissue, this maneuver includes the infected sternum.

Once the area is clean, the pectoralis major muscle is dissected on each side of the sternal area, raising the muscle flap, making the dissection in a practically avascular space, which is below the muscle and on the external surface of the thoracic wall, thus achieving advancement of the structures. At the top end, dissection is made until it reaches both clavicles, as for the lower end, it is possible by even raising the rectus abdominis during dissection of the pectoralis major´s caudal edge at the level of the xiphoid appendage, leaving the superior attachment of the rectus abdominis in its place. Laterally, the dissection shall be made by advancing the flap towards the mid-line and stopping when overlapping is achieved with both muscle borders without showing excessive tension, dissection is usually carried out at the level of the mid-clavicular line, or up to the anterior axillary line, ensuring irrigation of the flaps with the thoraco-acromial vascular pedicle, thus avoiding humeral injury at the muscular insertion and preventing ischemia of the pectoralis minor muscles. Once flaps are obtained, it is important to verify that the wound is clean and that residual sternum is with sufficient irrigation, then one or two drainages are left in the mediastinal space. [16] At that time, advancement of both flaps towards the mid-line is made, and overlapping their borders is done by placing one end onto the other, with a minimal overlap of 3 centimeters, suturing may be performed with simple "U" stitches (Figures 2 and 3), the recommended suture is frequently #1 vicryl, also non-absorbable #1 sutures may be used.

The space between the stitches must be maximum one centimeter apart without leaving any free space, giving the overlap more tightness, then two drainages are left below the overlapping muscular plane, one on each side of the dissected sites, then subcutaneous tissue is closed with absorbable suture, lastly the skin with 3-0 polypropylene.

The most frequent complications are: a) flap loss, b) dehiscence, c) persistence of the infectious process, d) hematomas, and e) functional shoulder movement problems. [14] Also to provide stability to the wall and prevent dehiscence after the surgery, it is prudent to use jockstraps or corsets to prevent lateral migration of the wound. Tailored (based on culture results) antibiotics must be maintained for four to six weeks, drainage rate should be revised every day to accomodate changes in management. [1]

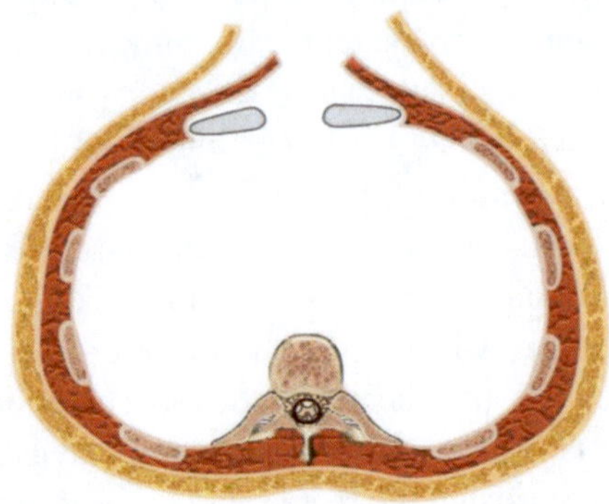

Figure 2. Axial view of the anterior thoracic wall with the pectoralis major dissected ready for overlapping.

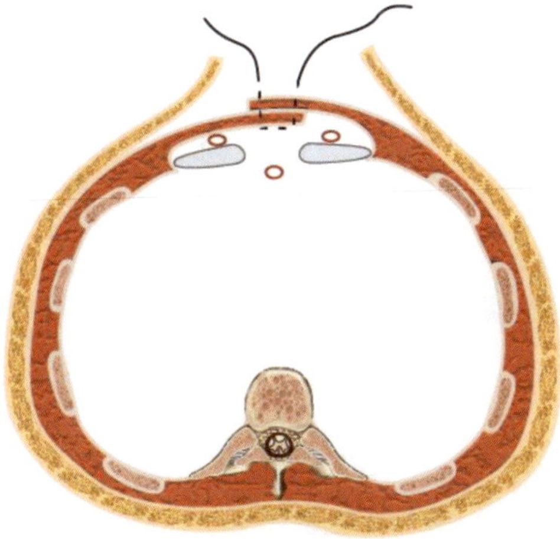

Figure 3. Axial view of the anterior thoracic wall when pectoralis major borders are overlapped and sutured with "U" stitches. Note the red circles are the site where the drains are placed.

Greater Omentum Lift (Omentoplasty)

Omentoplasty is another option to manage deep sternal wounds, either as a sole procedure, or as mentioned before, associated to pectoralis major muscles advancement procedure. Important properties of the omentum are its rich vascularity, angiogenic capacity, and immunologic properties; this benefit has been documented in the reconstruction of complex infected wounds. [18]

To do an omental lift, an incision (approximately 5-6 cm.) is made in the mid-line as a continuation of the sternotomy, dissection by planes is performed until reaching the abdominal cavity, then mobilization of the major omentum is done releasing it from its attachment to the transverse colon, the right gastroepiploic artery is dissected from the gastric wall and is split from its left counterpart at the level of the grater gastric curve, remembering that the stomach´s arterial supply will not be harmed, due to compensation from contralateral flow (Figure 4). Another way to obtain the flap is by not touching the gastroepiploic artery from both sides, and ligating it at its site of anastomosis (Figure 5).

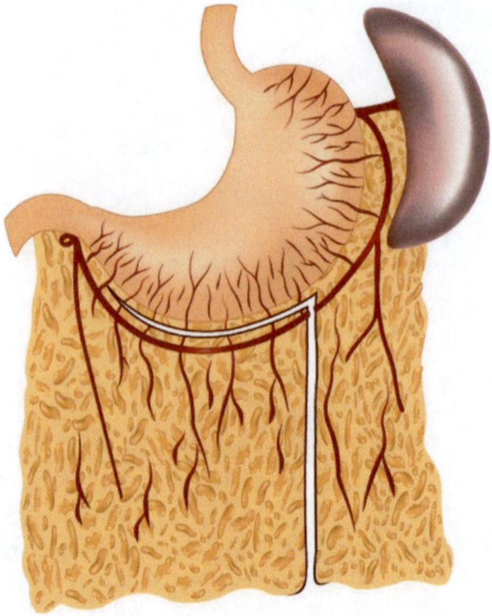

Figure 4. Schematic representation of omental flap by section of the grastroepiploic artery.

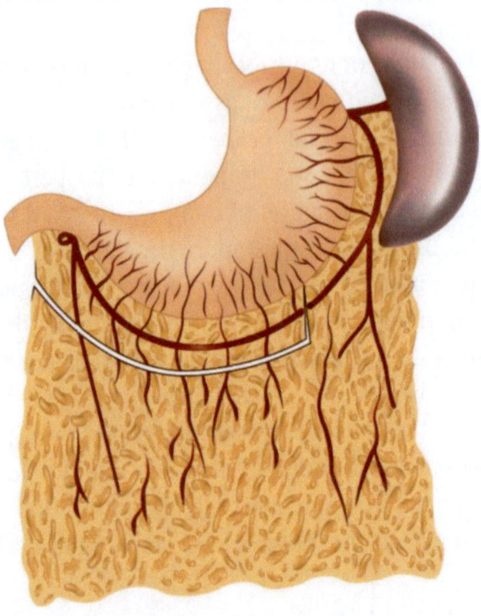

Figure 5. Schematic representation of omental flap without sectioning the gastroepiploic artery, only performed by ligating it (preserving gastric irrigation).

The omental flap (figure 6) is carried upwards to the thorax through an opening in the diaphragm, whereby entirely covering the space lost due to the dissected sternum (Figure 7). [18] Then, once the omental flap is in place, proceed to close the wound, if there is an important sternal loss, complement with advancement of the pectoralis major. The most frequent complications are: a) seromas, b) hematomas, c) flap tissue loss, d) abdominal cavity invasion (by infection), e) posterior wall hernias (very low frequency).

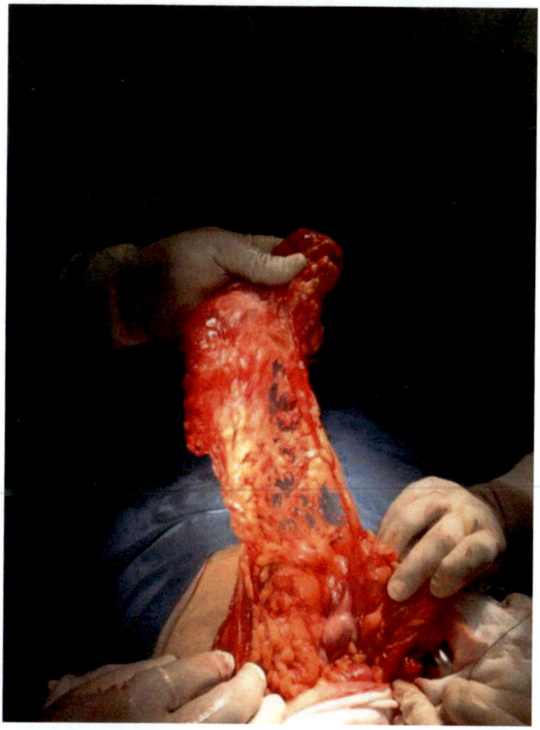

Figure 6. Omental flap once dissection is performed.

Negative Pressure Wound Therapy for Management of Post-Operative Mediastinitis

When an uncontrolled mediastinal infection is imminent, it is prudent to perform serial debridement and NPWT previous to the omentoplasty. This therapy, which is a closed system with negative pressure, was initially described by Davydov et al. [19] and developed in the United States in 1995 by Argenta et al. [20] It is formed of a polyurethane sponge with 400-600 μm pores which is placed on the wound, covered with an airtight transparent patch (drape), connected by a tubing system to a suction control computerized unit, in the mediastinum, a polyvinyl patch is cut-off and fitted to be placed within the wound under the sternum to protect vital structures, sterile gauze pads with petrolatum placed on the heart may also be used, creating an interface between them, then a second sponge is placed between the sternal edges and subcutaneous tissue.

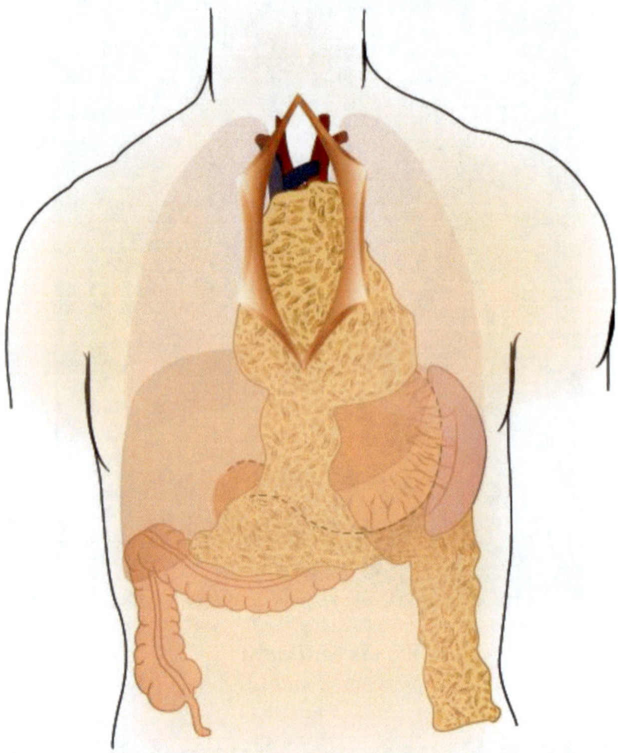

Figure 7. Schematic representation of the omental flap in its final place.

The unit is programmed at a negative pressure between 75-125 mmHg, said pressure acts intermittently for 2-5 minute periods (Figure 8). Once cultures are negative, the criteria to withdraw this therapy are also the absence of fever, normal serum C-reactive protein levels, and a clean macroscopic wound, as well as normal serum levels of white blood cells.

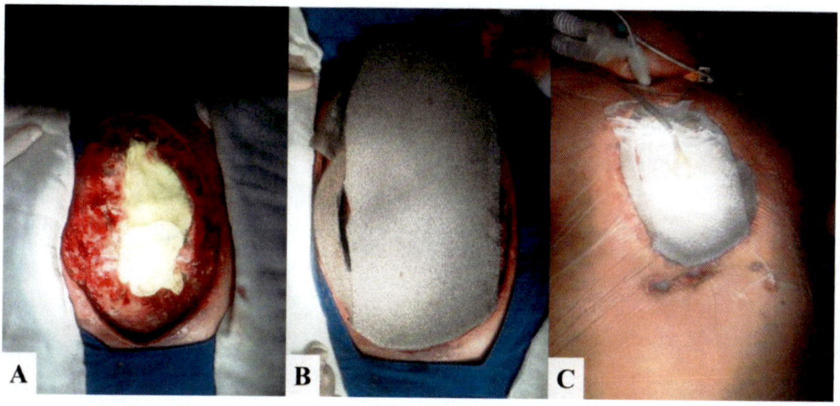

Figure 8. Steps for placement of the negative pressure wound therapy system, (A) a polyvinyl patch is cut and fitted on the heart to avoid injury from suction, then a polyutherane porous sponge goes on top, to finally complete the procedure with an adhesive transparent plastic drape connected by tubes to the computerized unit that controls intermittent negative pressure applied to the wound.

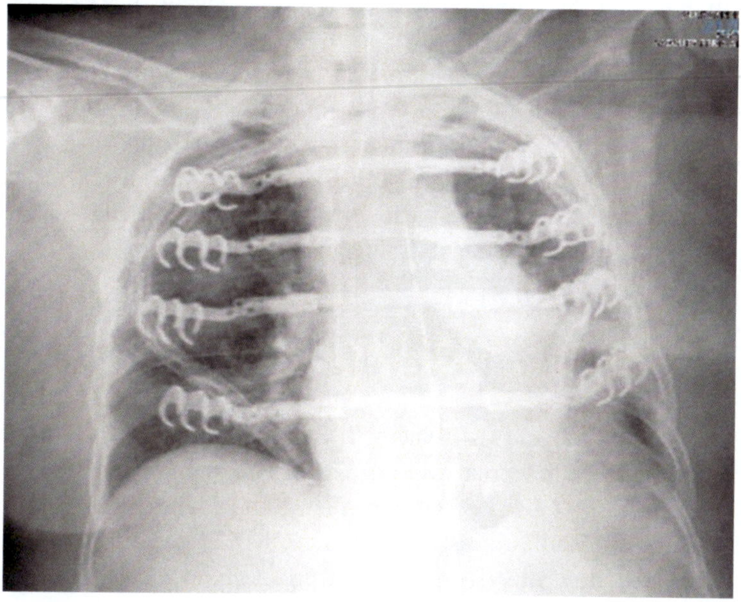

Figure 9. Titanium plates in position for anterior chest stabilization once the patient is without infection and a previous sternectomy was performed.

The therapy´s principle is to increment blood flow into the infected areas provoked by negative pressure, thus promoting infectious cleanup and granulation tissue generation, this increment in perfusion results in an augmented hydrostatic pressure gradient along the surrounding tissue arterioles. [21] A new suction system with negative pressure that also includes irrigation with sterile solution controlled by computer has also been used, which may produce successful results in a shorter period of time but requires more patients to demonstrate its effectiveness.

Also in some cases where NPWT alone has been unsuccessful, using it as an adjuvant therapy has become a viable option with overlapping pectoralis muscles advancement surgery, omentoplasty, rectus abdominis muscle flap, or as described for the sternum, osteosynthesis by means of horizontal titanium plates inserted in the parasternal spaces with consecutive sternal fixation (Figure 9). [19]

Conclusion

Post-operative mediastinal infections are a real catastrophe, as it was shown in the chapter, surgical options have the tendency to be extreme measures, and unfortunately simpler methods have not been devised yet, making this a continued challenge in these patients´ treatments. It is of the outmost importance that cardiac surgeons immediately identify superficial as well as other signs of infection in an effective manner so that the spread of disease is limited before other drastic decisions have to be made, such as omentoplasty or muscle advancement. Nonetheless NPWT sheds a light of hope in the future for the treatment of infected sternal wounds.

References

[1] Poncelet AJ, Langele B, Delaere B, Zech F, Glineur D. Algorithm for primary closure in sternal wound infection: a single institution 10-year experience. *Eur J Cardio-Thoracic Surg* 2008;33:232-238.

[2] The Parisian Mediastinitis Study Group. Risk factors for deep sternal wound infection after sternotomy: a prospective, multicenter study. *J Thorac Cardiovasc Surg* 1996;111:1200-1207.

[3] Borger MA, Rao V, Weisel RD, Ivanov J, Cohen G, Scully HE, David TE. Deep sternal wound infection: risk factors and outcomes. *Ann Thorac Surg* 1998;65:1050-1056.

[4] Penvi D, Mohr R, Lev-Run O, Locer C, Paz Y, Kramer A. Shapira influence of bilateral skeletonized harvesting on occurrence of Deep sternal wound infection in 1000 consecutive patients undergoing bilateral internal thoracic artery grafting. *Ann Surg* 2003;237:277-280.

[5] Garner JS, Jarvis WR, Emori TG, Horan TC, Hughes JM. CDC definitions for nosocomial infections. *Am J Infect Control* 1998;16:128-140.

[6] El Oakley RM, Wright JE. Postoperative mediastinitis: classification and management. *Ann Thorac Surg* 1996;61:1030-1036.

[7] Jurikiewicz MJ, Bostwick J III, Hester TR, Bishop JB, Craver J. Infected median sternotomy wound: successful treatment by muscle flaps. *Ann Surg* 1980;191:738-744.

[8] Colen LB, Huntsman WT, Morain WD. The integrated approach to suppurative mediastinitis: rewiring the sternum over transposed omentum. *Plast Reconstr Surg* 1989;84:936-941.

[9] Ringelman PR, Vander-Kolk CA, Cameron D, Baumgarther WA, Manson PN. Long-term results of flap reconstruction in median sternotomy wound infections. *Plast Reconstr Surg*1994;93:1208-1214.

[10] Belcher P, McLean N, Breach N, Paneth M. Omental transfer in acute and chronic sternotomy wound breakdown. *Thorac Cardiovasc Surg* 1990;38:186-191.

[11] Szerafin T, Jaber O, Péterffy A. Technical refinements of omentopexy and pectoralis myoplasty for poststernotomy mediastinitis. *Eur J Cardiothorac Surg* 2002;21:766.

[12] Robicsek F, Fokin A, Cook J, Bhatia D. Sternal instability after midline sternotomy. *Thorac Cardiovasc Surg* 2000;48:1-8.

[13] BrutusJ, Nikolis A, Perreault I, Harris P, Cordova C. The unilateral pectoralis major island flap, an efficient and straightforward procedure for reconstruction of full length sternal defects after postoperative mediastinal wound infection. *The British Association Plastic Surg*. 2004;57:803-805.

[14] Turgut O, Uraloglu M, Cagri A, Orbay H, Tekin F, Senzos O, Uraloglu G. Reconstruction of sternal defects with pectoralis major muscle flap. *Eur Plast Surg* 2008;30:223-228.

[15] Nestcher DT, Eladoumikdachi F, Goodman CM. Rectus abdominis muscle flaps used for median sternotomy wounds after ipsilateral internal mammary artery ligation. *Ann Plast Surg* 2001;47:223-228.

[16] Ascherman JA, Patel SM, Malhotra SM. Management of sternal wounds with bilateral pectoralis major myocutaneous advancement flaps in 114 consecutively treated patients: Refinements in technique and outcomes analysis. *Plast Reconstr Surg* 2004;114:676-683.

[17] Parissis H, AL-Alao B, Soo A, Orr D, Young V. Risk analysis and outcome of mediastinal wound and deep mediastinal wound infections with specific emphasis to omental transposition. *J Cardiothorac Surg* 2011;6:111.

[18] Baillot R, Cloutier d, Montalin L, Coté L, Lellouche F, Houde C, Gaudreau G, Voisine P. Impact of deep sternal wound infection management with vacuum assisted closure therapy followed by sternal osteosynthesis: a15-year review of 23,499 sternotomies. *Eur J Cardiothorac Surg* 2010;37(4):880-887.

[19] Tang at, Ohri SK, Haw MP. Novel application of vacuum assisted closure technique to the treatment of sternotomy wound infection. *Eur J Cardiothorac Surg* 2000;17:482-484.

[20] Argenta LC, Morkywas MJ. Vacuum-assisted closure: a new method for wound control and treatment: clinical experience. *Ann Plast Surg* 1997;38:563-576.

[21] Banwell PE. Topical negative pressure therapy in wound care. *J Wound Care* 1999;8:79-84.

In: Mediastinal Infections
Editor: Walid Leonardo Dajer-Fadel
ISBN: 978-1-63463-369-7

Chapter 11

Medical Management of Post-Operative Mediastinitis

***F. J. González-Ruiz*[1*] *and F. Baranda-Tovar*[1]**
[1]National Institute of Cardiology Ignacio Chávez, Mexico City, Mexico

Abstract

Median sternotomy allows surgeons an excellent access to mediastinal structures without discomfort associated to muscle-splitting incisions and rib retraction. Surgical site infection is not an extinct entity. The diagnosis of post-operative mediastinitis among patients with sternal wound complications is somewhat difficult, with and incidence rate of 1-4% but may show a mortality rate up to 45%. Risk factors for sternal instability are insulin-dependent diabetes mellitus, obesity, immunosuppressed state, chronic obstructive pulmonary disease, osteoporosis, history of renal failure, smoking and a malnourished state. Sometimes it is hard to treat, as fever, elevated C-reactive protein levels, and chest pain can be caused by general inflammatory reaction due to operative trauma and/or sternal dehiscence without infection. Hemodynamic monitoring and medical management of acquire a major relevance in high- risk patients and those suffering from comorbidities associated with hemodynamic instability, such as hemorrhage or septic shock.

* Correspondence: Francisco Javier González Ruíz, E-mail address: cardiocritmd@outlook.com.

In this chapter we will focus on the medical aspects involved in the management of critically ill patients with post-operative mediastinitis.

Introduction

Rationale for Hemodynamic Monitoring

The arguments to defend the use of specific types of monitoring techniques depend on evidence and prior experience using similar monitoring that was traditionally used and presumed to be beneficial, understanding the pathophysiology of the process being treated and documentation that the monitoring device, by altering therapy in otherwise unexpected ways, improves outcomes in terms of survival and quality of life. [1, 2]

On a philosophical level, one may consider monitoring of critically ill patients as serving a dual function. First, it can be used to document hemodynamic stability and the lack of need for acute interventions, and second, it can be used to monitor variables that vary from their defined baseline values. Therefore, knowing the limits that reflect actual physiological monitoring values is an essential aspect of its usefulness. [2]

On the physical side, hemodynamic monitoring can be invasive or noninvasive, and continuous or intermittent. Without any doubt, the choice of monitoring technique depends on the severity and comorbidities of the patient, so medical history and medical assessment are crucial. [2]

Post-operative mediastinitis (PM) monitoring should include body temperature, heart rate, systolic and diastolic arterial blood pressure, and respiratory frequency. Processed noninvasive variables include: electrocardiogram, transcutaneous pulse oximetry (SpO_2), expired CO_2, trans-thoracic echocardiography and non-invasive respiratory plethysmography. Most patients with mediastinitis may experience septic shock, and multiple comorbidities like dilated heart disease, poor ventricular function, active ischemia or cor-pulmonale; in this context, invasive monitoring should be placed for fluid management. Invasive hemodynamic monitoring of vascular pressure is usually performed by the percutaneous insertion of a catheter into a vascular space and transducing the pressure sensed at the distal end. This allows for continued monitoring and display of this complex pressure waveform. Similarly, intrapulmonary vascular catheters can be used to derive thermal signals and mixed venous oxygen (O_2) and saturation (SvO_2), needed to asses cardiac output and the adequacy of O_2 delivery, respectively. How useful this hemodynamic information is to diagnosis, treatment and prognosis is a function of its reliability, established treatment protocols, guidelines, and the physician's expertise, Tables 1 and 2 describe the measures that could be monitored during the post-operative period and the physiological relevance derived from monitoring. [2]

Table 1. Calculated measures using multiple measured variables including cardiac output by thermodilution, arterial blood gases and mixed venous blood gases. HR = heart rate, Ca O_2 = arterial oxygen content, Cv O_2 = mixed venous oxygen content, Pet CO_2 = end tidal carbon dioxide, SV = stroke volume

Calculated measures
Vascular resistances Total peripheral resistance : MAP/CO Systemic vascular resistance: (MAP-CVP)/CO Pulmonary arterial resistance: (Mean Ppa-Ppc)/CO
Vascular pump function Left ventricular stroke volume (SVIv)= CO/HR Left ventricular stroke work (SWIv)= (MAP-Ppao)/SVIv Preload-recruitable stroke work= SWIv/Ppao.
Oxygen transport and metabolism Global oxygen transport or delivery (DO_2)= CaO_2/CO Global oxygen uptake (VO_2)= (CaO_2-CvO_2)/CO Venous admixture. Ratio of dead space to total tidal volume (Vd/Vt)= $PaCo_2$/($PaCO_2$-$PetCO_2$)

Table 2. Possible monitored values during the post-operative period and their physiological interpretation

Invasive monitoring and its physiological relevance
Arterial pressure Mean arterial pressure (MAP) Organ perfusion inflow pressure Arterial pulse pressure and its variation during ventilation Left ventricular stroke volume changes and pulsus paradoxus. Preload responsiveness (if assessed during intermittent positive pressure ventilation. Arterial pressure waveform Aortic valvulopathy, input impedance, and arterial resistance. Used to calculate stroke volume by pulse contour technique.

Table 2. (Continued)

Invasive monitoring and its physiological relevance
Central venous pressure (CVP) Mean CVP If elevated, then effective circulating blood volume is not reduced. CVP variations during ventilation Tricuspid insufficiency, tamponade physiology. Preload responsiveness (if assessed during spontaneous breathing)
Pulmonary arterial pressure Mean pulmonary arterial pressure Systolic pulmonary artery pressure
Right ventricular pressure load. Diastolic pulmonary artery pressure and pulse pressure, and their variations during ventilation.
Right ventricular stroke volume, pulmonary vascular resistance Diastolic pressure tract changes in intrathoracic pressure during ventilation.
Pulmonary artery occlusion pressure. - Mean pulmonary artery occlusion pressure - Left atrial and left ventricular intraluminal pressure, and by inference, left ventricular preload. - Back pressure to pulmonary blood flow. - Pulmonary artery occlusion pressure waveform and its variation during occlusion and ventilation. - Mitral valvulopathy, atrial of ventricular etiology of arrhythmia, accuracy of mean pulmonary artery occlusion pressure to measure intraluminal left ventricle pressure, and pulmonary capillary pressure.

Why Measure Arterial Pressure?

Arterial pressure is the input pressure for organ perfusion. Organ perfusion is usually dependent on organ metabolic demand and perfusion pressure. With increasing tissue metabolism, organ blood flow proportionally increases by selective local vasodilation of low resistance arterioles. [2]

If cardiac output cannot increase as well, as in the case with heart failure, the blood pressure decreases, limiting the ability of local vasomotor control to regulate blood flow. If local metabolic demand remains constant, however, changes in arterial pressure are usually matched by changes in arterial tone so as to maintain organ blood flow relatively constant. This local vasomotor control mechanism is referred to as auto-regulation. Although auto-regulation occurs in many organs, such as the brain, liver, skeletal muscle, and skin, it is not a universal phenomenon. Thus, a normal blood pressure does not mean that all organs have an adequate amount of perfusion, because increases in local vasomotor tone and mechanical vascular obstruction can still induce asymmetrical vascular ischemia. [2]

Arterial Pressure Variations During Ventilation

The majority of the critically ill mediastinal surgical patients treated in the ICU are usually on mechanical ventilation. Mechanical ventilation induced arterial pressure variations have been described since antiquity as pulsus paradoxus. [3]

Recently a renewed interest in the hemodynamic significance of heart lung interactions has emerged. The commonly observed variations in arterial pressure and aortic flow seen during positive-pressure ventilation have been analyzed as a measure of preload responsiveness. [4]

The rationale for this approach is that positive-pressure ventilation-induced changes in either as systolic arterial pressure (used to describe pulsus paradoxus), arterial pulse pressure, or stroke volume can predict in which subjects cardiac output will increase in response to fluid resuscitation. Ventilation-induced changes in systolic arterial pressure (pulsus paradoxus) and arterial pulse pressure are easy to measure from arterial pressure recordings.

The greater the degree of systolic arterial pressure or pulse pressure variations over the respiratory cycle, the greater the increase in cardiac output in response to a defined fluid challenge. Recently, measuring the mean change in aortic blood flow during passive leg rising in patients with spontaneous breathing has also proven to be accurate in predicting preload responsiveness. [5]

Although arterial pressure variations are a measure of preload-responsiveness [6], the “traditional” preload measures, such as right atrial pressure, pulmonary artery occlusion pressure, end diastolic volume, and intrathoracic blood volume, poorly reflect preload responsiveness. [7]

Central Venous Pressure

Central venous pressure (CVP) has been used to monitor central venous blood volume and estimate right atrial pressure for many years, being wrongly used as a parameter and sometimes goal for replacement of intravascular volume in shock patients. The validity of this measure as an index of right ventricle preload is non-existent across numerous studies. It has been shown that CVP has a poor correlation with cardiac index, stroke volume, left ventricular end diastolic volume, and right ventricular end diastolic volume. [8-10]

Although a very high CVP demands a certain level of total circulating blood volume, one may have CVP of 20 mmHg and still have an underfilled left ventricle that is fluid responsive. In reported series, some patients who had low CVP failed to respond to fluid and some patients who had high CVP responded a fluid challenge. [11] Based on this and the poor correlation described above, it is impossible to define ideal values of CVP; however, there is evidence that volumes loading in patients who have CVP greater than 12 mmHg are very unlikely to increase cardiac output. [12] Thus, the only usefulness of CVP is to define relative hypervolemia, because an elevated CVP only occurs in disease.

Why Measure Pulmonary Artery Occlusion Pressure?

Pulmonary artery occlusion pressure in the context of patients with mediastinitis is used most often in the bedside assessment of: pulmonary vasomotor tone, intravascular volume status and left ventricular preload and performance.

Pulmonary circulation normally has a low resistance with pulmonary arterial diastolic pressure only slightly higher than pulmonary artery occlusion pressure, and mean pulmonary arterial pressure a few mmHg higher than pulmonary artery occlusion pressure.

Either and increased pulmonary vascular resistance or a passive pressure buildup from the pulmonary veins can induce pulmonary hypertension. If pulmonary hypertension is associated with an increased peripheral vascular resistance (PVR), then the causes are primarily within the lung. Diagnoses such as pulmonary embolism, fibrosis, essential hypertension or veno-occlusive disease have to be excluded. If PVR is normal, left ventricle (LV) dysfunction is the more likely cause of pulmonary hypertension. Regrettably, PVR poorly reflects true pulmonary vasomotor tone in diseased lungs and during mechanical ventilation, especially with the application of positive end-expiratory pressure (PEEP). [13]

Left Ventricular Preload

Pulmonary artery occlusion pressure is often taken to reflect LV filling pressure, and by inference, LV end diastolic volume. Patients who have cardiovascular insufficiency and a low pulmonary artery occlusion pressure are presumed to be hypovolemic and initially treated with fluid resuscitation, whereas patients who have similar presentation but an elevated pulmonary artery occlusion pressure are presumed to have impaired contractile function. Although there are no accepted high and low pulmonary artery occlusion pressures values for which LV under-filling is presumed to occur or not, pulmonary artery occlusion pressure values less than 10 mmHg are usually used as presumed evidence of a low LV end diastolic volume, whereas values greater than 18 mmHg suggest a distended LV. [14]

Mixed Venous Oxygen Saturation

SvO_2 reflects the pooled venous O_2 saturation, and is an important parameter in the assessment of the adequacy of DO_2, and its relation with global oxygen uptake (VO_2). A decrease of SvO_2 could be explained by a decrease in global oxygen transport (DO_2) or any of the parameters that determine this, such as SaO_2, cardiac output, and hemoglobin concentration, and also by an increase in VO_2.

A decrease of DO_2 will be followed by stable VO_2, with a consequent decrease of the SvO_2 until a critical value of DO_2 is reached where the tissue are no longer able to compensate having a constant VO_2, and VO_2 becomes dependent on DO_2 in an almost linear relation. At this level SvO_2, though continuing to decrease, becomes less sensitive to changes of tissue perfusion. [2]

SvO_2 measured from blood drawn from the distal tip of a pulmonary artery catheter represents the true mixed venous value of the blood blended in the right ventricle. Care must be taken to withdraw blood slowly, so that it does not get aspirated from the downstream pulmonary capillaries.

Superior vena cava O_2 saturation ($SvcO_2$) has evolved over the past years with the positive results of the Rivers et al., which demonstrated that in patients who had septic shock or severe sepsis admitted to the emergency department, and early aggressive resuscitation guided by $ScvO_2$, CVP, and mean arterial pressure (MAP) reduced 28 day mortality from 46.5% to 30.5%. [2]

Measures of SvO_2, however, remain the gold standard to reflect minimal O_2 delivery. Thus, using a defined threshold value for $ScvO_2$ to identify when to start or stop resuscitation in a critically ill patient is fundamentally flawed. Still, a loss in $SvcO_2$ (<65%) is invariably associated with a low SvO2 (<72%), making it less sensitive but sill clinically useful at lower threshold values. [2]

Hemodynamic Management

The hemodynamic management of patients with mediastinitis must focus on fluid management, antimicrobial therapy and cardiovascular stability. We will focus on critical ill patients and the recommendations must follow the international guidelines for management of patients with severe sepsis and septic shock.

Protocol must identify patients with recognized hypoperfusion (defined as hypotension persisting after initial fluid challenge or blood lactate concentration $\geq$ 4 mmol/L). During the first 6 hours, goals of initial resuscitation should include all of the following: CVP between 8 and 12 mmHg, MAP > 65 mmHg, urine output > 0.5 ml/kg/hr. and $SvcO_2$ or SvO_2 70 or 65%, respectively. Quantitative resuscitation improved survival rates with a 15.9% to 17.7% reduction in 28 day mortality rate. Surveillance on serum lactate should be done, every time both hypotension and serum lactate $\geq$ 4 mmol/L showed mortality rates around 46%. [15]

During the first 6 hours of resuscitation, if $SvcO_2$, less than 70% or SvO_2 equivalent or less than 65% persist with what is judged to be an adequate intravascular volume repletion in the presence of persisting tissue hypoperfusión, dobutamine infusion (to a maximum of 20 μg/kg/min) or transfusion of packed red blood cells to achieve a hematocrit of $\geq$ 30% in an attempt to achieve the $SvcO_2$ or SvO_2 are feasible options.

In mechanically ventilated patients or those with known preexisting decreased ventricular compliance, a higher target CVP of 12 to 15 mmHg should be achieved to account for the impediment of filling. Similar considerations may be warranted in circumstances of increased abdominal pressure. [15, 16, 17]

Elevated CVP may also be seen with preexisting clinically significant pulmonary artery hypertension, making use of this variable unreasonable for judging intravascular volume status. Although the cause of tachycardia in septic patients may be multifactorial, a decrease in elevated pulse rate with fluid resuscitation is often a useful marker or improving intravascular filling. [18]

The recommendation for initial fluid management are: in favor of crystalloids (grade IB) and against of hydroxyethyl starches for fluid resuscitation in severe sepsis and septic shock (grade IB). The guidelines suggest the use of albumin for resuscitating patients with severe sepsis and septic shock when they require substantial amounts of crystalloids (grade 2C). [15]

Two types of colloids are used in the peri-operative period for surgical patients: albumin (human derived) and hydroxyethyl starch (HES) synthetic solution. Crystalloid vehicles in which colloids are suspended may be isotonic 0.9% saline solutions of buffered (lactated/acetated) electrolyte solutions. HES solutions may be further grouped into older high molecular weight, high degree of molar substitution solutions (*hetastarch* dissolved in 0.9% or other carrier) versus modern lower molecular weight, and lower degree of molar-substitution solutions (*tetrastarch*). Although developed to enhance metabolism and elimination from the intravascular space thus improving safety versus older starches, modern tetrastarches, have shown to have significant risks in the intensive care unit setting. Whether HES is suspended in saline or in buffered electrolyte solution, patients with higher mortality risks at baseline are at particularly increased risk of renal injury even when resuscitated with modern starch solutions. On average, 42% of the nearly 7000 patients in the CHEST study were surgical patients, making it reasonable to extend findings to cardiac surgical patients. [19]

The pattern of kidney injury from tetrastarch use seems related to pinocytosis of metabolites into renal proximal tubular cells after glomerular filtration. Increase uptake into renal tissue occurs as plasma half life decreases with the newer starches *versus* the older starches. [19]

Starch-associated bleeding risk is not explained by hemodilution effects. Thromboelastographic differences are apparent consistent with impaired fibrin polymerization and decreased levels of factors VII, vWF, and XIII. [19]

Although used for decades in cardiac surgery patients, albumin may also have legitimate safety concerns. An increase in adverse outcomes with albumin use among patients with traumatic brain injury has been known for some time now. Impairment of the blood brain barrier in cardiac surgical patients is also now well described. Albumin is considerably more expensive and as a human derived product that carries a small but definite risk for the transmission of prions. Furthermore, even when viewed as a possible choice during goal direct therapy, the optimal type of fluid for preemptive volume optimization is actually unclear because randomized trials comparing crystalloids and albumin for goal directed therapy have not been conducted. Given the safe alternatives, it is also hard to defend the continued use of albumin. [19]

Respiratory Support

It is well known that sepsis and mediastinitis can cause an acute distress respiratory syndrome and have fatal consequences. In this context, recommendations for mechanical ventilation are: a 6 ml/kg. target of a tidal volume, use of predicted body weight, and plateau pressures should be measured in patients with acute respiratory distress syndrome (ARDS) and that the initial upper limit goal in a passively inflated lung be $\leq$30 cmH_2O. [15, 20]

The updated Berlin definitions describes ARDS as mild, moderate and severe (PaO_2/FiO_2 <300, <200 and <100 mmHg, respectively). Multiple studies have shown a decreased mortality in patients with a pressure-and-volume limited strategy for established ARDS. [21]

The largest trial of a volume-and-pressure limited strategy showed and absolute 9% decrease in all-cause mortality for patients with ARDS ventilated with tidal volumes of 6 ml/kg compared with 12 ml/Kg of the predicted body weight, and aimed for plateau pressures $\leq$ 30 cmH_2O. The use of lung protective strategies for patients with ARDS is supported by clinical trials and has been widely accepted.

No single mode of ventilation (pressure control, volume control) has consistently been shown to be advantageous when compared with any other that respect the same principles of lung protection. [21]

PEEP must be applied to avoid alveolar collapse at the end of expiration (atelectotrauma). As we know, raising PEEP in ARDS keeps lung units open to participate in gas exchange. This will increase PaO_2 when PEEP, is applied through either and endotracheal tube or a face mask. [22, 23, 24]

Three large multicenter trials using higher *versus* lower levels of PEEP in conjunction with low tidal volumes did not uncover benefit or harm. A meta-analysis using individual patient data showed no benefit in all patients with ARDS; however, patients with moderate or severe ARDS ($PaO_2/FiO_2 \leq 200$ mmHg) had decreased mortality with the use of higher PEEP, whereas those with mild ARDS did not. [25, 26, 27]

There are two recommended options for PEEP titration. One is to titrate PEEP (and tidal volume) according bedside measurements of thoraco-pulmonary compliance with the objective of obtaining the best values, reflecting a favorable balance of lung recruitment and overdistention. [28,29] The second is to titrate PEEP based on severity of oxygenation deficit and being guided by the FiO_2 required to maintain adequate oxygenation. [30, 31, 32]

A PEEP > 5 cmH_2O is usually required to avoid lung collapse [33]. The recruitment maneuvers in sepsis with severe refractory hypoxemia due to ARDS are suggested. In small trials, prone position demonstrated improved oxygenation, nevertheless associated with potentially life threatening complications, including accidental dislodging of endotracheal and chest tubes [34, 35, 36, 37]. Weaning protocols must be in place to evaluate spontaneous breathing and the ability to discontinue mechanical ventilation being satisfied by the following criteria:

An arousable hemodynamically stable (without vasopressor agents) patient, with no new potentially serious conditions, low ventilator and end expiratory pressure requirements and low FiO_2 requirements which ca be safely delivered with a face mask o nasal cannula.

There are extrapulmonary effects of mechanical ventilation that must be taken into consideration.

Adverse Cardiovascular Effects of Positive Pressure Ventilation

Positive-pressure ventilation can significantly change intra-thoracic physiological pressures. The extent of these changes depend on the amount of positive pressure applied to the airways and patient´s cardiopulmonary status. [38]

During inspiration with high tidal volumes (V_t) or when high levels of PEEP are used, the pulmonary capillaries that interlace the alveoli are stretched and narrowed. As a result, resistance to blood flow through pulmonary circulation increases. This increases right ventricular afterload. In normal healthy individuals, RV stroke volume is maintained in the face of increased pulmonary vascular resistance (PVR) because the RV contractile function is not severely impaired. However, in patients with compromised RV function, the RV cannot overcome these increases in PVR, and overdistension of the RV occurs, resulting in a decrease in RV output. [38] Dilation of the RV can also force the interventricular septum to move to the left. This phenomenon usually occurs when high airway pressure (P_{aw}) (> 15 cmH_2O) is used and the patient´s blood volume is depleted. When this happens, the left ventricle end diastolic volume (LVEDV) is encroached upon and left ventricle stroke volume may decrease because its ability to fill is limited. Septal shifting can significantly decrease cardiac output in patients with compromised LV function or in patients who are volume depleted. In the latter group, intravascular volume expansion may help to restore output from the left side of the heart by returning LV preload to normal.

The LV output may also be decreased when high V_T is used during positive pressure ventilation because the heart is compressed between the expanding lungs [38]. In addition to reduced venous return and ventricular function alterations, lower cardiac output may be caused by myocardial dysfunction associated with reduced perfusion of the myocardium and the resultant myocardial ischemia. The flow of blood into the coronary vessels depends on coronary perfusion pressure. The coronary artery perfusion pressure gradient for the LV is the difference between mean aortic diastolic pressure and left ventricular end diastolic pressure. A reduction in coronary arteries perfusion can result from any factor that decreases this pressure gradient. Thus, a reduction in cardiac output or blood pressure, coronary vasospasms, or direct compressive effect of the coronary vessels (caused by an increase in intrathoracic pressure during positive pressure ventilation) can decrease coronary perfusion and ultimately lead to myocardial ischemia. [38]

Effects of Lung and Chest Wall Compliance and Airway Resistance

Patients with very stiff lungs, such as those with ARDS or pulmonary fibrosis, are less likely to experience hemodynamic changes with high pressures because less of the alveolar pressure (P_{alv}) is transmitted to the intrapleural space. On the other hand, patients with compliant lungs and stiff (noncompliant) chest wall are more likely to have higher intrapleural pressures with positive pressure ventilation and experience more pronounced cardiovascular effects.

In patients with increased airway resistance (R_{aw}), even if peak pressures may are very high, much of the pressure is lost to the poorly conductive airways. As a consequence, high peak airway pressures may not be transmitted to the intrapleural space and the alveoli. [38]

Renal Effects of Mechanical Ventilation

It has been known for nearly half a century that pressurized breathing can induce changes in renal function. These changes can be divided into three areas:

- Renal response to hemodynamic changes resulting from high intrathoracic pressures.
- Humoral response, including antidiuretic hormone (ADH), atrial natriuretic factor (ANF), and renin-angiotensin-aldosterone changes occurring with positive pressure ventilation.
- Abnormal pH, $PaCO_2$, and PaO_2 that affect the kidneys.

Although urinary output stays fairly constant over a wide range of arterial pressures, it will become severely reduced as renal artery pressure decreases below 75 mmHg. Indeed, urinary output can actually stop in the presence of profound hypotension. Therefore, it would be reasonable to assume that the initiation of positive pressure ventilation would cause a decrease in cardiac output, which in turn would lead to a decrease in renal blood flow and glomerular filtration rates and ultimately a decrease in urine output. However, decreases in urine production seen during positive pressure ventilation (PPV) may not be caused entirely by a decrease in cardiac output because returning cardiac output to adequate levels is not accompanied by a proportional increase in urinary output.

Redistribution of blood flow inside the kidney may actually be an important factor that is responsible for changes in its function. [38]

Several different types of hormones may also influence urine output during mechanical ventilation. Specifically, these include ADH, ANF, and the renin-angiotensin-aldosterone cascade. Increases in the release of ADH, can reduce urine production by inhibiting free water excretion. The major determinant of ADH is the decrease of plasma osmolarity. Blood pressure reduction can also cause increased ADH release through the following mechanism. [38] Blood pressure changes during PPV may precipitate ADH release; the left atrium has volume receptors that send nerve impulses over a vagal pathway to the hypothalamus, which in turn can stimulate increases or decreases in ADH production and secretion. Baroreceptors in the carotid bodies and along the aortic arch sense changes in pressure that can also raise or lower ADH levels. Because both of these areas are exposed to intrathoracic pressure changes PPV can potentially affect ADH secretion. An interesting finding is that negative pressure ventilation inhibits ADH release and produces a diuretic effect, in contrast to PPV, which enhaces ADH release and result in oliguria. [38]

ANP is normally released when the atria are distended. PPV and PEEP can reduce the blood volume and stretch on the atria, they also can reduce atrial filling pressure by either causing mechanical compression of the atria or by decreasing right atrial stretch from low venous return. Reducing atrial stretch leads to decreased secretion of ANF. Reduced ANF levels contribute to water and sodium retention during PPV. [38]

Nutritional Complications during Mechanical Ventilation

Patients´ nutritional status must be carefully monitored and maintained if they are to recover from their illness and be weaned from mechanical ventilation. Both medical and surgical patients are subject to malnutrition during serious illness because of inadequate intake of food and increased metabolic rate associated with fever and wound healing. [38]

Furthermore, patients receiving ventilatory support are generally unable to have oral intake because of the endotracheal tube. Unless special routes for nutritional support are provided, such as nasogastric feeding or intravascular hyperalimentation, otherwise they will inevitably develop severe malnutrition. [38]

Nutritional depletion can cause several deleterious effects on patients, including reduction of their ability to maintain spontaneous ventilation from weakened respiratory muscles. It is important to understand that overfeeding can also lead to problems by increasing oxygen consumption, carbon dioxide production, and the need for increased expired minute ventilation, resulting in an increased work of breathing. [38]

The following are the malnourishment effects on mechanically ventilated patients:

- Reduced response to hypoxia and hypercapnia
- Muscle atrophy from prolonged bed rest and lack of use; includes respiratory muscle, especially if the patient is apneic and on controlled ventilation.
- Muscle waisting, including the respiratory muscle, from lack of nutrition.
- Respiratory tract infection from impaired cell immunity and reduced or altered macrophage activity.
- Decreased surfactant production and development of atelectasis.
- Reduced ability of the pulmonary epithelium to replicate, which slows healing of damaged tissue.
- Lower serum albumin levels, which affect colloid oncotic pressures and can contribute to pulmonary edema formation (colloid oncotic pressures < 11 mmHg with normal left atrial pressure).

Nutritional supplements should always be delivered by the most natural route possible. This means that oral feeding is the first choice, nasogastric feeding second, and catheters into the gastrointestinal tract third.

Early enteral nutrition has theoretical advantages in the integrity of gut mucosa and prevention of bacterial translocation and organ dysfunction, but also concerning is the risk of ischemia, mainly in hemodynamically unstable patients. [15, 39-43]. Although no consistent effect on mortality was observed, there is evidence that they benefit from some early enteral feeding on secondary outcomes, such as reduced incidence of infectious complications, reduced length of mechanical ventilation, and reduced ICU and hospital length of stay (LOS).

Clinical trials comparing full caloric early enteral feeding to lower targets in the critically ill have produced inconclusive results. Therefore, evidence is insufficient to support an early target of full caloric intake and, indeed with the existence of possible.

Underfeeding (60-70% of target) or trophic feeding (upper limit of 500 kcal) is probably a better nutritional strategy in the first week of severe sepsis/septic shock. The upper limit for trophic feeding is a somewhat arbitrary number, based in part that two recent studies used a range of 240-480 kcal. Underfeeding/trophic feeding strategies did not exclude advancing diet as tolerated in those who improved quickly. [15,44,45]

The trial by Casaer *et al.* reported that early initiation of parenteral nutrition led to longer hospital and ICU LOS, longer duration of organ supports, and higher incidence of ICU acquired infections.

Immune system function can be modified through alterations in the supply of certain nutrients, such as arginine, glutamine, or omega-3 fatty acid.

Arginine is a conditionally essential aminoacid like glutamine; much is derived from protein turnover and the remainder synthesized from citrulline in the kidney. Arginine has effects on creatine and collagen synthesis, modulation of lymphocyte proliferation and differentiation, cell growth and proliferation, wound healing, and insulin and glucagon secretion which is the sole precursor for nitric oxide synthesis.

However, arginine supplementation has generally been small and reported with variable effects on mortality, but the relevance of these findings in the face of potential harm is unclear. [15, 46, 47]

Glutamine is a conditionally an essential aminoacid, produced in large quantities by skeletal muscle, the brain and lungs. Studies of exogenous glutamine supplementation in critically ill patients have shown benefits related to anti-inflammatory roles, immune modulations, preservation of tissue function, and antioxidant capacity. Glutamine helps to maintain the gastrointestinal structure, reduces intestinal permeability and decreases the risk of bacterial translocation and development of infection. Supplementation has also been shown to attenuate cytokine release, preserve tissue function after sepsis, and attenuate insulin resistance. Provision of exogenous glutamine aids the body to increase protein synthesis, thereby improving wound healing and maintaining skeletal muscle mass. [47]

Some previous individual studies and meta-analyses showed positive secondary outcomes, such as reduction in infectious morbidity and organ dysfunction, but they are still unclear. Beneficial effects were found mostly in trials using parenteral rather than enteral glutamine.

Omega-3, Omega-6 fatty acids, or polyunsaturated fatty acids are not synthesized by the human body and must be obtained by dietary means or supplementation. These "essential fatty acids" are an integral part of the cellular membranes and serve as a substrate for the synthesis of mediators that regulate the intensity and duration of inflammation. Omega-3 polyunsaturated fatty acids can directly participate in inflammatory immune response by replacing omega-6 polyunsaturated fatty acid in the cellular membranes, therefore competing with arachidonic acid as a substrate for synthesis of less proinflammatory ecicosanoids and decreasing generation of inflammatory cytokines. [47]

Analgesia and Sedation

The general consensus supports the fact that limiting the use of sedation in critically ill ventilated patients can reduce the duration of mechanical ventilation, ICU and hospital LOS. The use of protocols for sedation is one method to limit sedative use, and a randomized controlled clinical trial found that protocolized sedation compared with usual care reduced the duration of mechanical ventilation, LOS, and tracheotomy rates.

Avoidance of sedation is another strategy, observational studies suggest that deep sedation is common in mechanically ventilated patients. Randomized controlled clinical trial found that the use of morphine boluses had significantly less need for ventilator support, shorter hospital and ICU LOS than patients who received sedation (propofol and midazolam) with morphine. Intermittent vs continuous methods for sedation delivery in critically ill patients have been also examined. Although no specific studies have been developed, the administration of intermittent sedation, daily sedative interruption, and systematic titration to a predefined endpoint, have demonstrated to decrease the duration of mechanical ventilation. In relation to neuromuscular blockade, they must be avoided if possible in septic patients without ARDS due to the risk of prolonged blockage following discontinuation. If these agents must be maintained, either intermittent bolus as required or continuous infusion with train-of-four monitoring of blockade depth should be used. [48]

Antibiotics

The microbial etiology of sternal wound infections is bacterial, both gram-negative and gram positive, in some occasions fungal. Staphylococcal species continue to be the most common offending organisms. Coagulase negative staphylococci have been reported to be one of the most significant pathogens during postoperative infections following cardiac surgery. When there are foreign material implants (used for surgery), coagulase negative staphylococci are known to play an important role. This is commonest when stainless steel wires are used for closure of the sternotomy during cardiac operations. Coagulase negative staphylococci has become the most significant organism in PM, accounting for 43% to 64% of all cases in recent studies. Antibiotic management requires testing for sensitivity, because *S. epidermidis* strains are frequently resistant to multiple antibiotics.

By far, *S aureus* remains the most common infectious agent responsible for PM. It may be more aggressive in nature and shows more classical signs of infection. This organism has been increasingly implicated in the colonization of nasal passages. It has been documented that the incidence of nasal colonization with *S aureus* in the normal population ranges from 10-15% and such colonization increases the risk of post-sternotomy mediastinitis.

Antimicrobial therapy should be administered as soon as the clinical suspicion of mediastinitis is evident, and simultaneously take blood cultures.

The administration of antibiotics should not delay surgical treatment, and antibiotic selection should be based on the institution´s prevalence of germs and must be adjusted as soon cultures results are obtained. [49]

Conclusion

The medical management of patients with mediastinitis encompasses a broad spectrum of issues that require skills and knowledge of the pathophysiological aspects surrounding the patient with this serious condition. A multidisciplinary approach is required, and the recognition of high risk patients should be identified in order to implement measures to reduce its appearance.

References

[1] Bellomo R, Pinsky MR. Invasive monitoring. In: Tinker J, Browne D, Sibbald W, editors. Critical care d standards, audit and ethics. London: Arnold Publishing Co., 2006. p. 82-104.

[2] Patricio M. Polanco MD, Michael R. Pinsky MD. Practical issues of hemodynamic monitoring at the bedside. *Surg Clin N Am* 2006;86:1431-1456.

[3] Rebuck AS, Read J. Assessment and management of severe asthma. Am *J Med* 1971;51(6):788–798.

[4] Michard F, Boussat S, Chemla D, Anguel N, Mercat A, Lecarpentier Y, Richard C, Pinsky MR, Teboul JL. Relation between respiratory changes in arterial pulse pressure and fluid responsiveness in septic patients with acute circulatory failure. *Am J Respir Crit Care Med* 2000;162(1):134–138.

[5] Monnet X, Rienzo M, Osman D, Anguel N, Richard C, Pinsky MR, Teboul JL. Passive leg raising predicts fluid responsiveness in thecritically ill. *Crit Care Med* 2006;34(5):1402–1407.

[6] Gunn SR, Pinsky MR. Implications of arterial pressure variation in patients in the intensive care unit. *Curr Opin Crit Care* 2001;7(3):212–217.

[7] Michard F, Teboul JL. Predicting fluid responsiveness in ICU patients: a critical analysis of the evidence. *Chest* 2002;121(6):2000–2008.

[8] Michard F, Alaya S, Zarka V, Bahloul M, Richard C, Teboul JL. Global end-diastolic volume as an indicator of cardiac preload in patients with septic shock. *Chest* 2003;124(5):1900–1908.

[9] Godje O, Peyerl M, Seebauer T, Lamm P, Mair H, Reichart B. Central venous pressure, pulmonary capillary wedge pressure and intrathoracic blood volumes as preload indicators in cardiac surgery patients. *Eur J Cardiothorac Surg* 1998;13(5):533–539.

[10] Buhre W, Weyland A, Schorn B, Scholz M, Kazmaier S, Hoeft A, Sonntag H. Changes in central venous pressure and pulmonary capillary wedge pressure do not indicate changes in right and left heart volume in patients undergoing coronary artery bypass surgery. *Eur J Anaesthesiol* 1999;16(1):11–17.

[11] Magder S, Georgiadis G, Tuck C. Respiratory variations in right atrial pressure predict-response to fluid challenge. *J Crit Care* 2004;7:76–85.

[12] Magder S. How to use central venous pressure measurements. *Curr Opin Crit Care* 2005;11(3):264–270.

[13] Abraham AS, Cole RB, Green ID, Hedworth-Whitty RB, Clarke SW, Bishop JM. Factors contributing to the reversible pulmonary hypertension of patients with acute respiratory failure studies by serial observations during recovery. *Circ Res* 1969;24(1):51–60.

[14] Forrester JS, Diamond G, Chatterjee K, Swan HJ. Medical therapy of acute myocardial infarction by application of hemodynamic subsets (first of two parts). *N Engl J Med* 1976; 295(24):1356–1362.

[15] Dellinger RP, Levy MM, Rhodes A, Annane D, Gerlach H, Opal SM, Sevransky JE, Sprung CL, Douglas IS, Jaeschke R, Osborn TM, Nunnally ME, Townsend SR, Reinhart K, Kleinpell RM, Angus DC, Deutschman CS, Machado FR, Rubenfeld GD, Webb SA, Beale RJ, Vincent JL, Moreno R; Surviving Sepsis Campaign Guidelines Committee including the Pediatric Subgroup. Surviving sepsis campaign: international guidelines for management of severe sepsis and septic shock: 2012. *Crit Care Med* Feb 2013;41(2):580-637.

[16] Levy MM, Dellinger RP, Townsend SR, Linde-Zwirble WT, Marshall JC, Bion J, Schorr C, Artigas A, Ramsay G, Beale R, Parker MM, Gerlach H, Reinhart K, Silva E, Harvey M, Regan S, Angus DC; Surviving Sepsis Campaign. The Surviving Sepsis Campaign: results of an international guideline-based performance improvement program targeting severe sepsis. *Crit Care Med* 2010;38(2):367-374.

[17] Bendjelid K, Romand JA. Fluid responsiveness in mechanically ventilated patients: A review of indices used in intensive care. *Intensive Care Med* 2003;29:352–360.

[18] Varpula M, Tallgren M, Saukkonen K, Voipio-Pulkki LM, Pettilä V. Hemodynamic variables related to outcome in septic shock. *Intensive Care Med 2005*;31:1066–1071.

[19] Shaw A, Raghunathan K. Fluid management in cardiac surgery: colloid or crystalloid? *Anesthesiology Clin* 2013;31(2):269–280.

[20] Franchi F, Silvestri R, Cubattoli L, Voltolini L, Mazzei MA, Giomarelli P. ARDS secondary to descending necrotizing mediastinitis treated by long-term extracorporeal respiratory support. *Respir Care* 2012;57(11):1970-1973.

[21] ARDS Definition Task Force, Ranieri VM, Rubenfeld GD, Thompson BT, Ferguson ND, Caldwell E, Fan E, Camporota L, Slutsky AS. Acute respiratory distress syndrome: the Berlin definition. *JAMA* 2012;307:2526–2533.

[22] Marini JJ, Ravenscraft SA. Mean airway pressure: Physiologic determinants and clinical importance–Part 1: Physiologic determinants and measurements. *Crit Care Med* 1992;20:1461–1472.

[23] Gattinoni L, Marcolin R, Caspani ML, Fumagalli R, Mascheroni D, Pesenti A. Constant mean airway pressure with different patterns of positive pressure breathing during the adult respiratory distress syndrome. *Bull Eur Physiopathol Respir* 1985;21:275–279.

[24] Pesenti A, Marcolin R, Prato P, Borelli M, Riboni A, Gattinoni L. Mean airway pressure vs. positive end-expiratory pressure during mechanical ventilation. *Crit Care Med* 1985;13:34–37.

[25] Mercat A, Richard JC, Vielle B, Jaber S, Osman D, Diehl JL, Lefrant JY, Prat G, Richecoeur J, Nieszkowska A, Gervais C, Baudot J, Bouadma L, Brochard L; Expiratory Pressure (Express) Study Group. Positive end-expiratory pressure setting in adults with acute lung injury and acute respiratory distress syndrome: A randomized controlled trial. *JAMA* 2008;299:646–655.

[26] Meade MO, Cook DJ, Guyatt GH, Slutsky AS, Arabi YM, Cooper DJ, Davies AR, Hand LE, Zhou Q, Thabane L, Austin P, Lapinsky S, Baxter A, Russell J, Skrobik Y, Ronco JJ, Stewart TE; Lung Open Ventilation Study Investigators. Lung Open Ventilation Study Investigators: Ventilation strategy using low tidal volumes, recruitment maneuvers, and high positive end-expiratory pressure for acute lung injury and acute respiratory distress syndrome: A randomized controlled trial. *JAMA* 2008;299:637–645

[27] Brower RG, Lanken PN, MacIntyre N, Matthay MA, Morris A, Ancukiewicz M, Schoenfeld D, Thompson BT; National Heart, Lung, and Blood Institute ARDS Clinical Trials Network. Higher versus lower positive end-expiratory pressures in patients with the acute respiratory distress syndrome. *N Engl J Med* 2004;351:327–336.

[28] Briel M, Meade M, Mercat A, Brower RG, Talmor D, Walter SD, Slutsky AS, Pullenayegum E, Zhou Q, Cook D, Brochard L, Richard JC, Lamontagne F, Bhatnagar N, Stewart TE, Guyatt G. Higher vs lower positive end-expiratory pressure in patients with acute lung injury and acute respira-tory distress syndrome: Systematic review and meta-analysis. *JAMA* 2010;303:865–873.

[29] Amato MB, Barbas CS, Medeiros DM, Schettino Gde P, Lorenzi Filho G, Kairalla RA, Deheinzelin D, Morais C, Fernandes Ede O, Takagaki TY. Beneficial effects of the "open lung approach" with low distending pressures in acute respiratory distress syndrome. A prospective randomized study on mechanical ventilation. *Am J Respir Crit Care Med* 1995;152(6 Pt 1):1835–1846.

[30] The Acute Respiratory Distress Syndrome Network. Acute Respiratory Distress Syndrome Network: Ventilation with lower tidal volumes as compared with traditional tidal volumes for acute lung injury and the acute respiratory distress syndrome. *N Engl J Med* 2000; 342:1301–1308.

[31] Mercat A, Richard JC, Vielle B, Jaber S, Osman D, Diehl JL, Lefrant JY, Prat G, Richecoeur J, Nieszkowska A, Gervais C, Baudot J, Bouadma L, Brochard L; Expiratory Pressure (Express) Study Group. Expiratory Pressure (Express) Study Group: Positive end-expiratory pressure setting in adults with acute lung injury and acute respiratory distress syndrome: A randomized controlled trial. *JAMA* 2008;299:646–655.

[32] Meade MO, Cook DJ, Guyatt GH, Slutsky AS, Arabi YM, Cooper DJ, Davies AR, Hand LE, Zhou Q, Thabane L, Austin P, Lapinsky S, Baxter A, Russell J, Skrobik Y, Ronco JJ, Stewart TE; Lung Open Ventilation Study Investigators. Lung Open Ventilation Study Investigators: Ventilation strategy using low tidal volumes, recruitment maneuvers, and high positive end-expiratory pressure for acute lung injury and acute respiratory distress syndrome: A randomized controlled trial. *JAMA* 2008;299:637–645.

[33] Gattinoni L, Caironi P, Cressoni M, Chiumello D, Ranieri VM, Quintel M, Russo S, Patroniti N, Cornejo R, Bugedo G. Lung recruitment in patients with the acute respiratory distress syndrome. *N Engl J Med* 2006;354:1775–1786.

[34] Stocker R, Neff T, Stein S, Ecknauer E, Trentz O, Russi E. Prone positioning and low-volume pressure-limited ventilation improve survival in patients with severe ARDS. *Chest* 1997;111:1008–1017.

[35] Lamm WJ, Graham MM, Albert RK. Mechanism by which the prone position improves oxygenation in acute lung injury. *Am J Respir Crit Care Med* 1994;150:184–193.

[36] Jolliet P, Bulpa P, Chevrolet JC. Effects of the prone position on gas exchange and hemodynamics in severe acute respiratory distress syndrome. *Crit Care Med* 1998;26:1977–1985

[37] Guerin C, Gaillard S, Lemasson S, Ayzac L, Girard R, Beuret P, Palmier B, Le QV, Sirodot M, Rosselli S, Cadiergue V, Sainty JM, Barbe P, Combourieu E, Debatty D, Rouffineau J, Ezingeard E, Millet O, Guelon D, Rodriguez L, Martin O, Renault A, Sibille JP, Kaidomar M. Effects of systematic prone positioning in hypoxemic acute respiratory failure: A randomized controlled trial. *JAMA* 2004;292:2379–2387.

[38] Cairo JM. Pilbeam's mechanical ventilation. Physiological and clinical Applications. *Fifth Edition Page*. 316-324.

[39] Moore EE, Jones TN. Benefits of immediate jejunostomy feeding after major abdominal trauma–A prospective, randomized study. *J Trauma* 1986;26:874–881.

[40] Chiarelli A, Enzi G, Casadei A, Baggio B, Valerio A, Mazzoleni F. Very early nutrition supplemen tation in burned patients. *Am J Clin Nutr* 1990;51:1035–1039.

[41] Eyer SD, Micon LT, Konstantinides FN, Edlund DA, Rooney KA, Luxenberg MG, Cerra FB. Early enteral feeding does not attenuate metabolic response after blunt trauma. *J Trauma* 1993;34:639–643.

[42] Minard G, Kudsk KA, Melton S, Patton JH, Tolley EA. Early versus delayed feeding with an immune-enhancing diet in patients with severe head injuries. *J Parenter Enteral Nutr* 2000;24:145–149.

[43] Nguyen NQ, Fraser RJ, Bryant LK, Burgstad C, Chapman MJ, Bellon M, Wishart J, Holloway RH, Horowitz M. The impact of delaying enteral feeding on gastric emptying, plasma cholecystokinin, and peptide YY concentrations in critically ill patients. *Crit Care Med* 2008;36:1469–1474.

[44] Rice TW, Mogan S, Hays MA, Bernard GR, Jensen GL, Wheeler AP. Randomized trial of initial trophic versus full-energy enteral nutrition in mechanically ventilated patients with acute respiratory failure. *Crit Care Med* 2011;39:967–974.

[45] National Heart, Lung, and Blood Institute Acute Respiratory Distress Syndrome (ARDS) Clinical Trials Network, Rice TW, Wheeler AP, Thompson BT, Steingrub J, Hite RD, Moss M, Morris A, Dong N, Rock P. Trophic vs full enteral feeding in patients with acute lung injury: The EDEN randomized trial. *JAMA* 2012;137:795–803.

[46] Bertolini G, Iapichino G, Radrizzani D, Facchini R, Simini B, Bruzzone P, Zanforlin G, Tognoni G. Early enteral immunonu trition in patients with severe sepsis: Results of an interim analysis of a randomized multicentre clinical trial. *Intensive Care Med* 2003;29:834–840.

[47] Hayes GL, McKinzie BP, Bullington WM, Cooper TB, Pilch NA. Nutritional Supplements in Critical Illness. *AACN Adv Crit Care* 2011;22(4);301-316.

[48] Barr J, Fraser GL, Puntillo K, Ely EW, Gélinas C, Dasta JF, Davidson JE, Devlin JW, Kress JP, Joffe AM, Coursin DB, Herr DL, Tung A, Robinson BR, Fontaine DK, Ramsay MA, Riker RR, Sessler CN, Pun B, Skrobik Y, Jaeschke R; American College of Critical Care Medicine. Clinical Practice Guidelines for the Management of Pain, Agitation, and Delirium in Adult Patients in the Intensive Care Unit. *Crit Care Med* 2013;41(1):263-306.

[49] Engelman R, Shahian D, Shemin R, Guy TS, Bratzler D, Edwards F, Jacobs M, Fernando H, Bridges C; Workforce on Evidence-Based

Medicine, Society of Thoracic Surgeons. The Society of Thoracic Surgeons practice guideline series: antibiotic prophylaxis in cardiac surgery, part II: antibiotic choice. *Ann Thorac Surg* 2007;83:1569–1576.

[50] Tammelin A, Hambraeus A, Ståhle E. Mediastinitis after cardiac surgery: improvement of bacteriological diagnosis by use of multiple tissue samples and strain typing. *J Clin Microbiol* 2002;40(8):2936-2941.

In: Mediastinal Infections
Editor: Walid Leonardo Dajer-Fadel
ISBN: 978-1-63463-369-7

Chapter 12

Chronic Mediastinitis

W. L. Dajer-Fadel[1*]
[1] Cardiothoracic Surgery Department, General Hospital of Mexico
"Dr. Eduardo Liceaga", Mexico City, Mexico

Abstract

Chornic mediastinitis is a rare disorder that encompasses multiple etiologies; they could be due to granulomatous processes, such as histoplasmosis, syphilis, tuberculosis, coccidoidomicosis and sarcoidosis, as well as non-granulomatous diseases. It is caused by proliferation of acellular collagen and fibrous tissue within the mediastinum. It has been also associated to immunologic processes or foreign bodies that were not removed. Symptoms are generally associated to compression of vital structures such as the superior vena cava, pulmonary arteries and veins, or major airways; expressed as wheezing, dyspnea, cough, chest pain, dysphagia and hemoptysis. Simple chest X-rays could suggest the diagnosis, however, a contrast enhanced CT is the tool of choice to properly evaluate these cases, more so when vascular structures are affected. The role of surgery is generally palliative, it is usually performed to diagnose or to relieve compromised structures from a mass effect to alleviate symptoms of compression.

[*] Correspondence to: Walid Leonardo Dajer-Fadel, E-mail address: drdajer@gmail.com.

Introduction

Fibrosing mediastinitis was first described by Nathan Oulmont in 1855. [1] As seen in other chapters, treatment of mediastinal infections are troublesome and this is not the exception; the chronic –fibrosing- type is a rare disorder caused by invasive proliferating tissue within the mediastinum that develops in a matter of years, compressing vital structures which eventually lead the patient to seek medical attention. Symptoms related to superior vena cava syndrome (SVCS) are very common, where dyspnea is the earliest sign, followed by cough, chest pain, dysphagia, cyanosis, congestion, headache and dizziness. [2] In other cases, where pulmonary artery compromise is imminent, patients arrive with shortness of breath and chronic cough, eventually, due to retrograde vascular compromise; also signs related to SVCS are evident. [3] When major airways are affected, compressions of these structures are evident when atelectasis ensues with a mixture of the clinical findings mentioned above. The chapter will be presented as a short review of the major causes of chronic mediastinitis; their diagnostic criteria and treatment protocols will be discussed.

Granulomatous Causes

Histoplasmosis: Several reports indicate *Histoplasma capsulatum* as a cause of this disease. It is usually associated with a previous granulomatous disease; eventually mediastinal fat is replaced with fibrous tissue. Infection with this fungus has been estimated to be 40 million in the United States, with 500 000 new cases occurring every year; [4] most of the time these are self-limiting, however, <1% result in this complication. A large proportion is found in the United States in the regions of Kentucky and the Southeast. [5, 6] The exact pathophysiologic mechanism is unknown; damage is believed to be due to antigen-mediated inflammation and infiltrative fibrosis. [7] Clinically, a patient with any of the symptoms described above, that in imaging studies appears with perihilar calcifications especially in chest CTs, it is most likely to be affected with a histoplasmosis mediastinitis. As an adjunct, bronchoscopy could be a valuable tool in the diagnostic work-up. Manali et al. found that tracheobronchial concentric narrowing, severe hyperemia, and mucosal edema are usually found when visualizing the airways. [8] Operative resection is indicated when compromise of vital structures are evident, However the use of steroid therapy (most effective when patients have high serum IgG4) has proven to reduce symptoms and improve the clinical picture. [9, 10]

Tuberculosis: This is another cause known to produce fibrosing mediastinitis, it is usually due to mediastinal lymphatic growth that compresses the structures within it, provoking caval compression, obliteration of main and intermediary right lobar bronchus, also the left airways may be affected, and hemoptysis are common signs. In occasions, anti-tuberculous treatment is not enough making management troublesome. [2, 11]

Coccidoidomycosis: An infection caused by *Coccidioides immitis,* a soil inhabiting fungus, common in the Southwest dessert of the United States including the state of Arizona, symptomatic in 40% of patients, with 1% to 10% of severe complicated cases, very rarely presents as mediastinitis, usually in a chronic pattern, but it can also progress to a septic state being fatal. In occasions, anti-fungal treatment is not effective, so surgical treatment may be warranted, however, information on the subject is so scarce that more cases need to be documented for an optimal approach to be suggested. [12-14]

Non-Granulomatous Causes

Behçet disease: A rare immune-mediated small-vessel systemic vasculitis often diagnosed by mucous membrane ulceration and ocular problems. Only three reports exist in the literature causing mediastinal involvement, generally seen with SVCS often associated with thrombosis, however, in chronic mediastiadinitis this syndrome could be caused by a mass effect on the superior vena cava; also it has been described as an abnormal reaction to *Histoplasma capsulatum* that could lead to a fibrosing mediastinitis. [15-17]

Methylsergide: A medication used for the treatment of migraine, has been reported to cause effects on the mediastinum such as mediastinal fibrosis. Saxena et al. [18] reported a case of a 60-year old male presented with angina and coronary artery compromise due to thickening of the aortic wall, after surgery, a biopsy revealed sclerosing mediastinitis. Very few reports address this cause but it should always be taken into account.

Radiologic Imaging

As mentioned before, most of the time, patients will visit a hospital when symptoms are evident, by this time, unfortunately, the growing mediastinal fibrosis has already caused compressive effects on viscera, X-rays will almost always diagnose a mediastinal mass, however a contrast-enhanced CT is warranted to determine exactly at which part is this hyperdense lesion compressing, mediastinal lymph nodes should be analyzed with precision and evaluate if any of these invade airways (as seen in tuberculosis) or vascular structures; it also helps having it as a topographical reference when surgical treatment is planned. Finally, to accurately evaluate pulmonary function, a ventilation-perfusion scan helps to properly follow patients throughout their disease, or as said before, plan the optimal approach for resection.

Conclusion

Fibrosing chronic mediastinitis has various causes, the chapter reviewed (although scarce) the most common of them, other etiologies have been reported, but only as isolated cases without much importance to the author´s point of view. It is imperative that the physician performs a very thorough history and physical to suspect the disease, backed by excellent radiological images, and decide whether to follow up on the patient with medical treatment, or perform a surgical resection to alleviate their symptoms.

References

[1] Oulmont, N (1855)Des Oblitérations de la veine cave supérieure. J.B. Ballière. Paris, France.

[2] Fijołek J, Wiatr E, Błasińska-Przerwa K, Roszkowski-Sliz K. Fibrosing mediastinitis as an untypical complication of tuberculosis: case report. *Pol Arch Med Wewn* 2009;119(11):752-755.

[3] Guerrero A, Hoffer EK, Hudson L, Schuler P, Karmy-Jones R. Treatment of pulmonary artery compression due to fibrous mediastinitis with endovascular stent placement. *Chest* 2001;119(3):966-968.

[4] Gurney JW and Conces DJ. Pulmonary histoplasmosis. *Radiology* 1996;199:297–306.

[5] Loyd JE, Tillman BF, Atkinson JB and Des Prez RM. Mediastinal fibrosis complicating histoplasmosis. *Medicine (Baltimore)* 1988;67:295–310.

[6] Murray JF, MillsJ. Pulmonary infectious complications on human immunodeficiency virus infection [review] *Part II Am Rev Respir Dis* 1990;141:1582-1598.

[7] Goodwin RA, Nickell JA, Des Prez RM. Mediastinal fibrosis complicating healed primary histoplasmosis and tuberculosis. *Medicine* (Baltimore) 1972;51:227-246.

[8] Manali ED, Saad CP, Krizmanich G, Mehta AC. Endobronchial findings of fibrosing mediastinitis. *Respir Care* 2003;48(11):1038-1042.

[9] Inoue M, Nose N, Nishikawa H, Takahashi M, Zen Y, Kawaguchi M. Successful treatment of sclerosing mediastinitis with a high serum IgG4 level. *Gen Thorac Cardiovasc Surg* 2007;55(10):431-433.

[10] Ichimura H, Ishikawa S, Yamamoto T, Onizuka M, Inadome Y, Noguchi M, Sakakibara Y. Effectiveness of steroid treatment for hoarseness caused by idiopathic fibrosing mediastinitis: report of a case. *Surg Today* 2006;36(4):382-384.

[11] Galván MF, Portal JA, Gorarredona MP, Izquierdo LG. Fibrosing mediastinitis mimicking sarcoidosis. *Clin Respir J* 2014. doi: 10.1111/crj.12107.

[12] Ampel NM, Mosley DG, England B, Vertz PD, Komatsu K, Hajjeh RA. Coccidioidomycosis in Arizona: increase in incidence from 1990 to 1995. *Clin Infect Dis* 1998;27:1528-1530.

[13] Louie L, Ng S, Hajjeh R, et al. Influence of host genetics on the severity of coccidioidomycosis. *Emerg Infect Dis* 1999;5:672-680.

[14] Rady MY, Lopez A, Patel BM, Larson JS. Pyo-mediastinitis: A complication of pulmonary coccidioidomycosis. *Can J Infect Dis* 2003;14(3):170-172.

[15] Kanne JP, Mohammed TL. Fibrosing mediastinitis associated with Behçet's disease: CT findings. *Clin Radiol* 2007;62(11):1124-1126.

[16] Harman M, Sayarlioglu M, Arslan H, Ayakta H, Harman E. Fibrosing mediastinitis and thrombosis of superior vena cava associated with Behçet's disease. *Eur J Radiol* 2003;48(2):209-212.

[17] Abid R, Hadj Taieb Abid F, Chaabane M, Boussen K, Robbana A, Bouhaouala H, Ber Maiz H, Hamza R. [Superior caval syndrome caused by chronic mediastinitis in Behçet's disease]. *J Radiol* 1995;76(2-3):155-157.

[18] Saxena P, Tesar PJ. Mediastinal fibrosis causing myocardial ischemia. *Ann Thorac Surg* 2005;80(6):2368-2370.

EDITOR'S CONTACT INFORMATION

Dr. Walid Leonardo Dajer-Fadel, M.D.,
Cardiothoracic and Minimally Invasive Thoracic Surgery
Cardiothoracic Surgery Department,
General Hospital of Mexico Dr. Eduardo Liceaga.
Ave. Cuauhtemoc 403 ed. 12 ap.102 Col. Roma Sur,
Mexico City, Mexico 06760
Tel: +525512861038
Email: drdajer@gmail.com

Index

A

B

C

D

E

H

I

M

N

P

R

S

V

Y

Z